The Wellness & Prevention Paradigm

ALSO BY JAMES L. CHESTNUT

The 14 Foundational Premises for the Scientific and Philosophical Validation of the Chiropractic Wellness Paradigm

The Innate Diet & Natural Hygiene

Innate Physical Fitness & Spinal Hygiene

The Innate State of Mind & Emotional Hygiene

Available at www.thewellnesspractice.com

The Wellness & Prevention Paradigm

Dr. James L. Chestnut
B.Ed., M.Sc., D.C., C.C.W.P.

"I take it for granted, when I am invited to lecture anywhere, for I have had a little experience in that business, that there is a desire to hear what I think on some subject, though I may be the greatest fool in the country, and not that I should say pleasant things merely, or such as the audience will assent to; and I resolve, accordingly, that I will give them a strong dose of myself. They have sent for me, and engaged to pay me, and I am determined that they shall have me, though I may bore them beyond all precedent. So now I would say something similar to you, my readers."

Henry David Thoreau – *Life Without Principle*

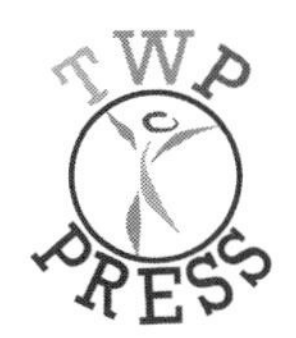

Victoria, British Columbia, Canada

Notices:

Published in 2011 by TWP Press,
431 Durban Street, Victoria, B.C. V8S 3K2

Chestnut, Dr. James L.
The Wellness & Prevention Paradigm
Revolutionary discoveries from the fields of genetics, lifestyle and health can save lives, save money, and save healthcare.

Includes bibliographical references.

Library Archives Canada
ISBN: 978-0-9868264-0-5

Printed and bound in the United States

DEDICATION

I dedicate this book to saving the millions of lives, trillions of dollars, and crumbling healthcare systems that are caused by preventable illnesses and their ineffective treatments. I dedicate this book to evidence-based change. I dedicate this book to all healthcare practitioners, regardless of profession, who devote themselves to improving patient health outcomes. I dedicate this book to those with the humility to admit changes are necessary, the honesty to investigate what these changes are, and the integrity to implement these changes into practice.

ACKNOWLEDGEMENTS

There are few times when the phrase 'would not have been possible' has literal meaning in an acknowledgement in a book. This is one of those rare times. Without the assistance, guidance, moral support, sweat equity, devotion, emotional investment, and dedication to a shared mission contributed by Dr. Richard Baxter, finishing this book on time would not have been remotely possible. I simply could not ask for a better friend, colleague, editorial consultant, doctor, techy nerd, or mentor. You are important and appreciated Rick. Thank you for your sacrifices, they were neither insignificant nor unrecognized. I could not ask for a better Bob Cratchit to my Scrooge. Next year there will be coal on the fire and a few days off!

My blessings certainly do not end with Dr. Baxter. Dr. Keith Milne, another colleague I am also privileged to call a friend, worked tirelessly, and I'm sure what felt endlessly, on the images, diagrams and bibliography. Thanks Keith, and please forgive the intrusion into your holiday time.

As deadlines came and went, pressure grew, and the window of opportunity to meet printing deadlines shrank, my father, Dr. C.W. Chestnut, generously offered his decades of experience correcting manuscripts as a professor. Thanks Dad, and you're welcome for the opportunity to correct my work with a green light and free conscience!

Most of all I am excited to acknowledge my wonderful family - my wife Lori and my children Meghan and Tyson. I thank them for their support and their sacrifices. They share me with my mission and they do so with encouragement, patience, and understanding. They also share my mission with me; for this I am eternally blessed and eternally grateful.

Lori and I just recently got married. To give you an idea of her level of support and understanding, I was away lecturing the two weekends prior to our wedding and the weekend after we got married. That was a busy month, for both of us of course. I wrote and read a poem for the wedding which I think expresses how I feel as well as I am able.

On our Wedding, at our River, with our Children, Forming our New Family

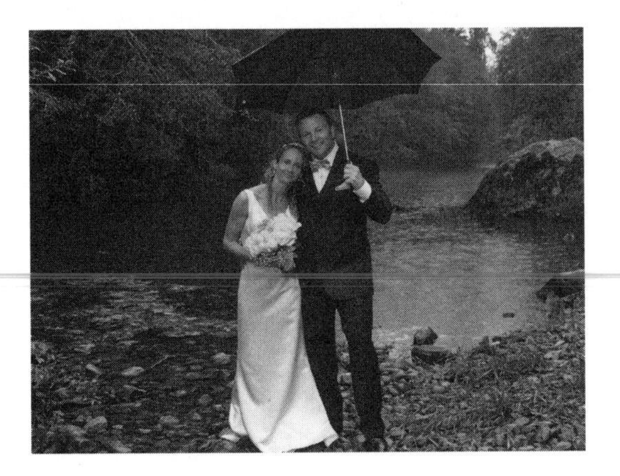

A seed planted with a chance passing of neighbors in similar situation, germinated with a few passing words, and sprouted as words became conversation.
It grew with your gift of Christmas cookies for a single father and his daughter,
an Easter Egg hunt grew roots, and it blossomed with the smiles of our children, and their laughter.

A hug, a blunderous airline travel bag re-gift, a first date,
a shaving lip laceration that made me so late.
An East Sooke trail birthday hike, the bond was sealed,
the first I love you, my heart revealed.

It was inevitable, it had to take place,
our first run together, no chance to save face.
Up Sinclair, up Tolmie, up Wedgewood we run,
me struggling on my own, you pushing Tyson!

Few nights without children, not what either of us would endeavor,
parents first, lovers second, now a family forever.
We took our time and allowed our children to see,
what a wonderful thing it is, to create a loving family.

The universal law of the family tree remains intact,
you can always add, but never subtract.
So we are Tyson and Lori plus Meghan and James,
a marriage of four, now all Chestnut in name.

A more fortunate family you will never meet,
even though we avoid sugar, dairy, and wheat.
A healthy family we have vowed to make,
but please dear guests, be careful, don't get between our kids and the cake!

Now some words for you Tyson my extraordinary son,
I'm so proud of you, you are so strong, so kind, and so handsome.
You are strong, yet gentle, and you have such a unique special power,
you can sleep anywhere, in any position, no matter the hour!

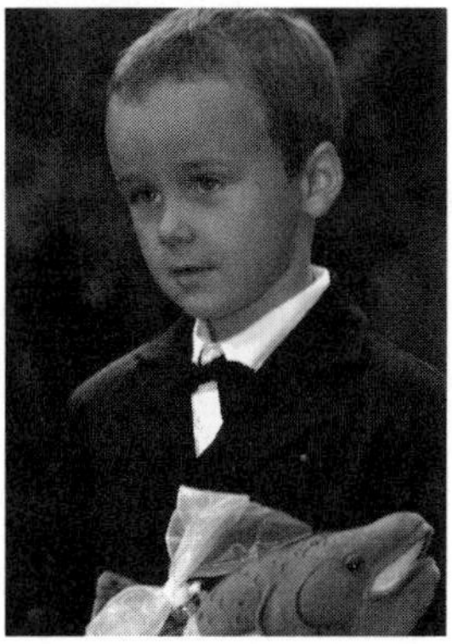

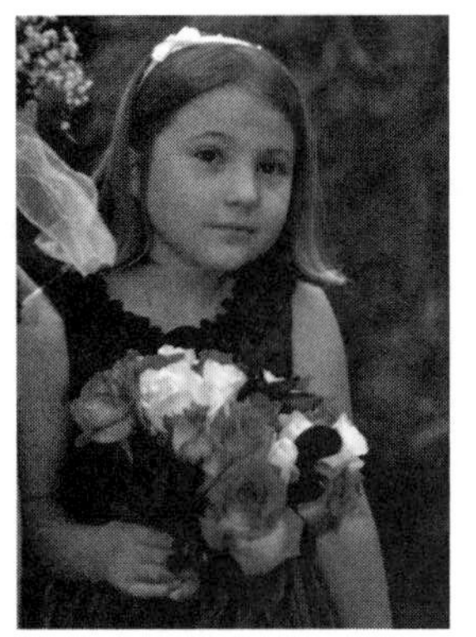

My Meghan, my bubba, with your champion's heart,
you are so strong, so beautiful, so brave, and so smart.
Although perfect to me, there is one flaw with you my Meg,
you were born with a giant, empty dessert leg!

Now back to you my beautiful bride,
the one I adore and respect, and will soon call my wife with such pride.
I love you Lori, and I make this public decree,
for the rest of our lives I will always strive to make you feel safe, loved, appreciated, and important to me.

I often teach that FALLING in love is about desire,
and wanting to be with someone we respect and admire.
But what KEEPS us in love, and what makes a love real,
is how the one we love, about ourselves, makes us feel.

So here now, at our river, before our family, friends, and you,
I make this solemn vow to you Lori, and promise it to be true.
I will spend the rest of our lives together,
whether I am at home or lecturing afar,
doing all I know how, to make you feel wonderful about who you are.

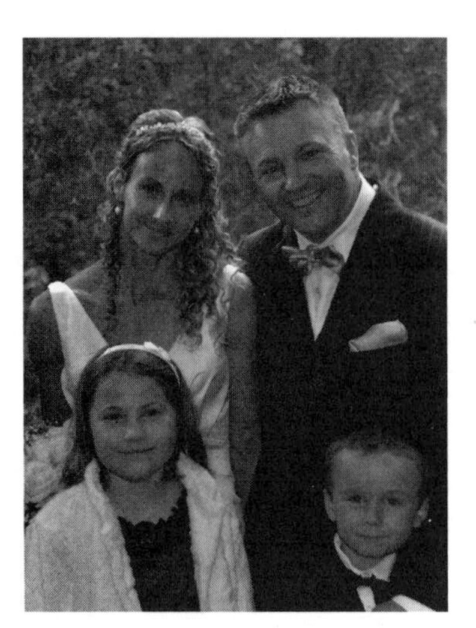

You are my hero, my best friend, my sunshine, and my life.
Thank you so much my love, for becoming my wife.

FOREWORD

I met Dr. Chestnut in 1996, when we were first year students at chiropractic college. It soon became clear to me that this was an individual who took nothing at face value. As with any post-secondary professional program, the sheer volume of course work caused most of our class, including me, to adopt a policy of "don't ask any questions, just learn the material as it is presented." Dr. Chestnut, on the other hand, set himself apart by asking countless questions that usually started with "how" or "why" and virtually always ended with "where did you read that, may I have a copy". I was one of many who were taught by him that this was the only way to determine if the material being taught in lectures, or contained in textbooks, was supported by valid evidence or merely based on accumulated opinion and dogma.

When he and I decided to work together after graduation I knew that this dedication to investigation and truth-seeking would continue, and so it has for the past ten years. I have observed the same relentless pursuit of the truth applied with equal vigor to clinical decision-making in the context of an individual patient; or in the broader scope of how best to answer the questions posed in this book. Time and time again I have witnessed him resist the temptation of the expedient or popular choice and adhere to his core value of doing the right thing, even if it meant adding more time demands onto an already full schedule. Often I have heard Dr. Chestnut asked what motivates him to spend so much time travelling, teaching, researching, and writing. He will give his own answer to this question in the introduction and throughout this book. Please do not confuse his use of the term "mission" with the trite use of it as a marketing tactic by so many other individuals, businesses, and corporations. As I often tell the attendees at our seminars, with dedicated effort you might be able to match the amount of time Dr. Chestnut spends reading and researching but you would be hard pressed to catch up to all the time he HAS spent in the past. When he says he is on a mission, he means it and he inspires those of us around him to take up the cause. As the saying goes, the tide raises all boats. Dr. Chestnut has raised a lot of boats. Like the respected generals of history, he is one of those people who truly "leads from the front". I came across the following quote the other day that seems to sum it up quite nicely, so many thanks to Mr. Marley for providing these appropriate words:

"The people who are trying to make this world worse are not taking the day off. Why should I?"

Bob Marley

Five years ago, Dr. Chestnut offered me the privilege and responsibility of assisting him in teaching some of the components of the wellness lifestyle certification program that he created and developed. Much of the material contained in this book has been gathered throughout the process of developing and constantly updating this program. As you read this book you may decide that some of the concepts presented are "nothing new". This was not the case five to ten years ago. In fact, it was quite bold to suggest some of these very same concepts. What has been most remarkable to me is that, in the entire time that I have been teaching this material, I have never had to admit that any of the fundamental concepts were flawed. Unlike fads or gimmicks, which can just as easily be discredited as they can be promoted, this material has withstood the test of time. One of the main reasons why is because it has been based on science and tested by reason and logic. In fact, it is now common for me to see and hear material on television and in the popular press that supports the concepts that Dr. Chestnut presented years ago.

You might ask how it is possible that one person could have come up with such simple yet powerful ideas and concepts. I will explain from my privileged vantage point of having seen much of this material being developed. Dr. Chestnut possesses a rare combination of skills: a scholar's intellect, a parliamentarian's willingness to debate, a mathematician's logic, a child's voracious appetite for information and knowledge, and a bulldog's persistence. It is difficult to pose a question that he has not already asked and answered. You will see this as you read through the content of this book. You will also see that he has not spent his time in the laboratory conducting primary research. His passion and skill has been to take that information which already exists from a wide variety of fields and synthesize it into a single holistic explanatory model. Perhaps even more importantly, he makes the complicated simple and understandable. As you will see in the very deliberate relaxed writing style of this book, Dr. Chestnut is much more interested in having his audience understand than having his audience muse about how learned or intelligent he is.

I am reminded of the character in the Patch Adams movie that advises Dr. Adams to, "Look past the problem. See the solution. See what no one else sees. See what everyone chooses not to see... out of fear, conformity or laziness." This has been, in my opinion, Dr. Chestnut's defining talent. Hans Selye summarizes such a talent even more eloquently when he says:

"It is not to see something first, but to establish solid connections between the previously known and the hitherto unknown that constitutes the essence of scientific discovery. It is this process of tying together which can best promote true understanding and real progress."

Hans Selye

I hope that, as you read this book, you will come to explore a new paradigm and be open to honestly critiquing the beliefs and opinions you have held about health and healthcare. I also implore you to read this book right through to the final chapter. Just as you will learn about the effects of your lifestyle choices; the knowledge you gain by reading the content of this book will also accumulate. By the time you reach the last page, you will have been introduced to many concepts that work synergistically and holistically with each other. Furthermore, each page contains one or more pieces of information that will empower you to be the one in charge of your health. The benefit you gain will be directly proportional to the extent that you understand and adopt the practices contained herein.

You will also notice that the margins have been enlarged and a sample question has been included on almost every page. This has been done to prompt you to become an active reader, or as Dr. Chestnut likes to say, an informavore. As the text stimulates new thoughts and ideas use the remaining space to write your own questions. Once you have finished reading this book, I suggest that you pass it along to someone you love. It could very well be the greatest gift you have ever given them.

Richard A. Baxter, B.Eng., D.C.

CONTENTS

Introduction

"Cowardice asks the question, 'Is it safe?'
Expediency asks the question, 'Is it politic?'
And Vanity comes along and asks the question,
'Is it popular?'
But Conscience asks the question, 'Is it right?'
And there comes a time when we must take
a position that is neither safe, nor politic, nor
popular, but we must do it because Conscience
tells us it is right."

Martin Luther King, Jr.

I have written this book because over the past 25 years I have gathered information which I feel a moral obligation to share. I have written this book because I care. I have written this book as part of my mission to save the millions of lives and trillions of dollars which I can prove are being lost due to preventable illness.

As a species humans are facing our greatest threat in history. That threat is chronic illness. The Black Plague killed 30 percent of Europe. Chronic illness is now killing 80 percent of the industrial world.[1] Humans are now the sickest species on earth. We have gone from super species to sickest species in less than a century. Never in history has a species suffered with so much illness, with so much cancer, diabetes, heart disease, obesity, and other chronic illness.

The research is unequivocal; we are in the midst of a chronic illness pandemic that threatens not only our health but the very fabric of our society and the very existence of our species. We are, literally, the sickest species on the planet. We have the sickest children, the sickest teenagers, the sickest adults, and the sickest elderly in the history of our species - in the history of any species. Over half of our entire industrial population has a chronic illness and over 80 percent of our adult industrial population has chronic illness. Chronic illness is the leading cause of death and suffering; 80 percent of our population is dying and will die from chronic illness.[2] Despite ever increasing medical spending and medical procedures the rates of chronic illness have been steadily rising for over 50 years. **The current system is not working. We don't need more debate about who should pay for healthcare, we need to start debating about what kind of healthcare we should pay for.**

Over 80 percent of our workforce has chronic illness. Chronic illness is responsible for 9 days of absenteeism per employee per year and up to 91 days of lost productivity per employee per year.[3] Chronic illness is the leading cause of personal, corporate, and government debt and bankruptcy. By 2017 chronic illness will cost 4.3 trillion dollars per year in the U.S. alone.[4] This represents $12 billion per day, $500 million per hour, and over 8 million dollars per minute – EVERY DAY. The U.S. is NOT an outlier. On a per capita basis, these figures apply to most developed nations.

Imagine what this means for large employers like the government or large corporations. Imagine that you have 1,000,000 employees and 800,000 of them have a chronic illness (55 percent of them have two or more chronic illnesses). Imagine that you not only have to pay for their medical costs but you also have to pay their wages even when they are not at work.

In fact, you not only have to pay for their wages when they are absent, you also have to pay for the wages of the people you bring in to replace them. Further, you also have to pay full wages for up to another 91 work days that are lost due to their decreased productivity because of their chronic illness. Think about this for a second. Most employees get four to six weeks paid holidays per year. In addition to this, if they have chronic illness, they also get paid for another 12 weeks of non-working days per year. This makes a total of up to 18 weeks or over 4 months of paying wages for no productivity.

Don't forget that on top of this there are the medical costs of the drugs and surgeries that are associated with the standard medical treatment of chronic illness. Does anyone honestly think this is sustainable for employers or employees? Does anyone actually believe that any business with 8 out of 10 chronically ill employees can compete with a business that has healthy employees? The scenario is even worse for small business. Imagine if you only have 10 employees and 8 of them have chronic illness. Worse, imagine you run your own business and you are your only employee and you have chronic illness. This is not a labour versus employer issue. Chronic illness is unsustainable at all levels from individual to corporation to government to society.

Chronic illness is *lifestyle illness*. Chronic illness rates have risen exponentially since 1900, as have prescription drug use and surgery. Our genes have not undergone any significant change during this period of time. It can't be genes. During this period of exponential increase in chronic illness our genes have remained virtually unchanged but our *lifestyle has changed significantly.* The changes in our lifestyle away from what we genetically require as a species mirror the increases in chronic illness.

We are NOT simply detecting more illness and thus skewing the data regarding chronic illness incidence. Obesity and diabetes alone, which are causal factors in virtually every other chronic illness, have increased exponentially in just the last two decades. Detecting obesity and diabetes is NOT technology dependent; it requires a scale and perhaps a tool to measure body fat percentage or body mass index and a simple blood sugar test. This is NOT new technology.

We are NOT simply living longer and thus inevitably developing more chronic illness. The percentage of the population aged 65 or older did not increase at all between 1990 and 2010 so aging has nothing to do with the per capita increases in chronic illness rates or expenditures.[5] Further, chronic illness rates and drug prescription rates are rising most rapidly in our children and in middle aged adults. Half our children are overweight and each year more have diabetes, asthma, and attention and behavior issues.[6] Our elderly have much higher rates of illness than the elderly in non-industrial cultures. Our children have much more chronic illness than the children in non-industrial cultures. Our elderly and our children today have exponentially more chronic illness than our elderly and our children did only a generation ago. Lifespan has not significantly changed in this time. [7]

The *only* solution to the pandemic of chronic illness, and the pandemic of human suffering and financial burden that it causes, is *fewer sick people.* The only way to achieve a society with fewer sick people is to correctly answer the two most important questions regarding the health of our citizens.

These questions are: **"Why are we getting so sick?" and**

"What do we need to do to get and stay well?" I have devoted the last 25 years, virtually all my adult life, to finding answers to these two questions. Finding answers to these questions, and discovering why traditional medical researchers and clinicians have failed to correctly answer these questions, has been the sole purpose of my professional life, and a large part of my personal life. Sharing the answers to these questions is the purpose of this book. These answers can save millions of lives and trillions of dollars. These answers can save businesses and governments and societies and these answers are the ONLY way we will be able to create meaningful reform and save healthcare.

The answers to these questions are self-evident when you ask the right questions.

We need to stop asking what chronic illnesses we have and how to treat them (diagnosis and treatment) and start asking why we are developing chronic illnesses and how to avoid them (wellness and prevention).

We are sick because we have changed our lifestyle patterns away from what our species requires to genetically express health and toward what causes us to genetically express chronic illness. The only way we can get and stay well is to change our lifestyle patterns back to what is genetically suitable for our species. The reason traditional medical researchers and clinicians have not answered these questions correctly is not due to a lack of intelligence or a lack of caring or a lack of effort. It is due to the paradigm that guides traditional medical research and clinical intervention. It is due to the fact that the entire traditional medical system operates within a gene-centric Sickness & Treatment Paradigm that is inaccurate regarding the cause of illness and the source of health. Until this gene-centric Sickness & Treatment Paradigm is replaced with the more accurate lifestyle-centric Wellness and Prevention Paradigm the correct answers to the two most important questions will never be found and the chronic illness pandemic and the unsustainable human, economic, and societal burdens it causes will never be eradicated.

The fact is that the single greatest determinant of whether you will get sick or get and stay well IS YOUR LIFESTYLE CHOICES. This is an INDISPUTABLE FACT. Once it is understood that how we eat, move, think and interact is the cause of chronic illness, the fact that changing these behaviors is the only viable option to prevent and/or recover from chronic illness becomes self-evident. The FACT is that the only way to create a society with fewer sick people and more healthy people is to adopt lifestyle behaviors that are genetically congruent, that promote the genetic expression of health, and prevent the genetic expression of unsustainable adaptation, fatigue, and illness.

The FACT is that no drug or surgery will EVER be the wellness and prevention solution for illnesses caused by malnutrition or overeating or the ingestion of toxins in our foods. No drug or surgery will EVER be the wellness and prevention solution for problems caused by sedentary living or poor physical fitness. No drug or surgery will EVER be the wellness and prevention solution for problems caused by lack of self esteem, lack of life satisfaction, or lack of positive attitudes, thoughts, emotions, and social relationships.

This book is about revealing the truth and exposing the falsehoods regarding why humans have become so sick. This book is about explaining why the current diagnosis and treatment approach has not worked, why it will never work, and what we need to implement in the future that has already been proven to work. The survival of our species, our way of life, our economy, our standard of living and of our planet depend on this change. This book is dedicated to eliciting this change.

Chapter 1
The Biology of Health and Sickness

"I have always felt that the only trouble with scientific medicine is that it is not scientific enough. Modern medicine will become really scientific only when physicians and their patients have learned to manage the forces of the body and the mind that operate via vis medicatrix naturae (the healing power of nature)."

Rene Dubos

Are humans separate from nature?

Let me take you on a little bit of a journey explaining how I discovered the right questions to ask regarding health and sickness. I am the son of a Ph.D. biologist. I spent my childhood in the wilderness. I grew up on a hobby farm where we grew vegetables, had fruit trees, kept animals, and worked and played physically every day (more play than work for me, as my parents will happily tell you). Growing up on a farm and spending so much time studying and living in natural environments shaped me, it gave me a naturalist paradigm or belief system; it made me a lifelong biophiliac (a lover of nature).

Let me give an example of how things are different in a naturalist paradigm. You know the ten second rule that states if something drops on the ground and you pick it up quickly you can still eat it? We had about a ten day rule, there just wasn't a lot of fuss and muss about germs, a bit of dirt, or animal dung. We grew up knowing that the chemicals used to clean were far more dangerous than the natural bugs and dirt that were found in a natural environment. If we got sick (which was exceedingly rare), we didn't run for a pill, instead we tried to figure out why we got sick, we rested, ate healthy foods and drank lots of water. We were not afraid of an egg with chicken dung on it, we were horrified by bleached white eggs with pale yolks that had no flavor. It was just different. It was just natural. I grew up in that paradigm.

The thing that most significantly shaped my paradigm, the

thing that has allowed me to deliver this life changing message all over the world, is that, from a very early age, I realized that I was not outside of the ecosystem of the planet looking in. I understood that I was part of the ecosystem, not separated from it, or in control of it, or smarter than it. From as early as I can remember I had a sense of awe and respect for ecosystems; they were the source and governing systems of the nature that I loved so much. Most of my holidays, in fact virtually every holiday I ever went on, were trips deep into the wilderness. My father and I regularly went fishing or on horseback trips into the mountains. We built cabins and used them year after year. I could probably fly fish before I could walk. My dad probably untangled my fishing reel a thousand times. It was only after I became a father myself that I realized how much this must have affected his "relaxing" fishing trips. I would never accuse my father of being a patient man but when I think of all those tangles I realize he turned into the biblical Job on fishing trips. Thanks Dad.

Now, there was something else that fundamentally shaped my belief systems (my paradigm) and my life. During the short time span that I was a child, from when I was three years old to the time I was a teenager, I saw the environment around me dramatically change. When I was a young child, there were rivers that I couldn't put my line in without catching a fish in minutes. The rivers were surrounded by old growth forest and the forests were full of wildlife; full of deer, and bears, and owls, and eagles and cougars and insects. By the time I was a teenager, many of these paradises had changed dramatically. There were no fish left, there was no forest left, and the animals had disappeared.

Is our environment getting healthier or sicker?

I can remember going to mountain lakes that were so beautiful and so pristine that even as a child it would take my breath away. Tragically, by the time I was a teenager they had been completely destroyed. I couldn't find a tree, only stumps and garbage left by the logging companies. I remember crying, even as a child, because I was devastated to see this, not because I couldn't catch any fish but because the animals had been so harmed and so devastated. I've always tried to imagine what it must have been like for native peoples to watch as the forests and rivers and lakes they had lived in harmony with for generation upon generation were destroyed by the European settlers. It really is so tragic. We could have done it so much better, so much more sustainably, with so much more kindness and compassion and common sense. Sigh.

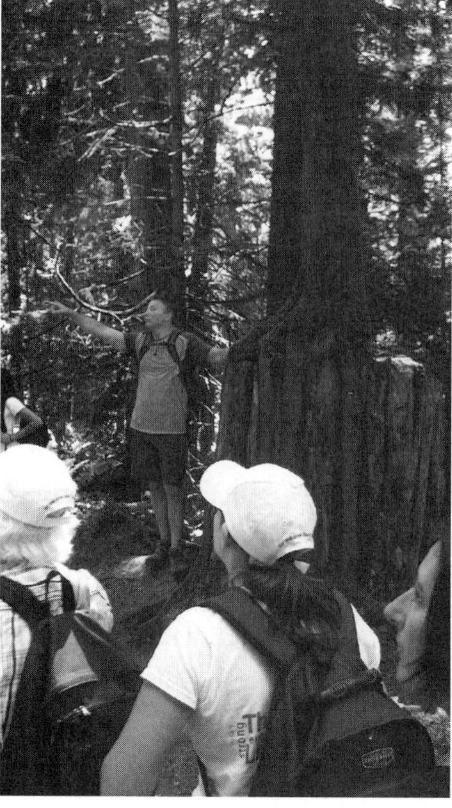

So when I first embarked on this journey, I was really much more of an environmentalist or a conservationist than I was a humanist. My concern when I grew up was mostly for wild animals. I loved wild animals and, to be honest, I had developed a dislike and distrust of humans, at least the domesticated, industrialized humans. I would drive anybody who would listen crazy with facts about animals, or asking them about animal facts. I think that, unlike many conservationists who really only want to save fish and deer so they can have things to catch or hunt later, I actually wanted to save animals for the sake of the animals and the trees for the sake of the trees. Even today when I lead my 3 day Eat Well – Move Well – Think Well Innate Lifestyle™ Implementation camps I love to gather the group around my favorite trees and rivers and trails so they can experience the same sense of awe and wonder that I do.

Do humans need healthy ecosystems?

They do experience this, by the way, to a person, at every camp. The participants are completely moved by the experience of feeling like they are part of the ecosystem. If you are interested in attending one of these camps you can get more information at www.thewellnesspractice.com. It is truly a life changing experience for everyone involved. Even the camera crew that was filming for the upcoming documentary had life changing experiences!

I always did, and still do, have a feeling of respect and admiration for plants and animals and for nature.

I don't worship nature, I am just profoundly grateful for it and feel a deep sense that I am part of it and it is a part of me. Biologically (and metaphysically) speaking of course, this is accurate.

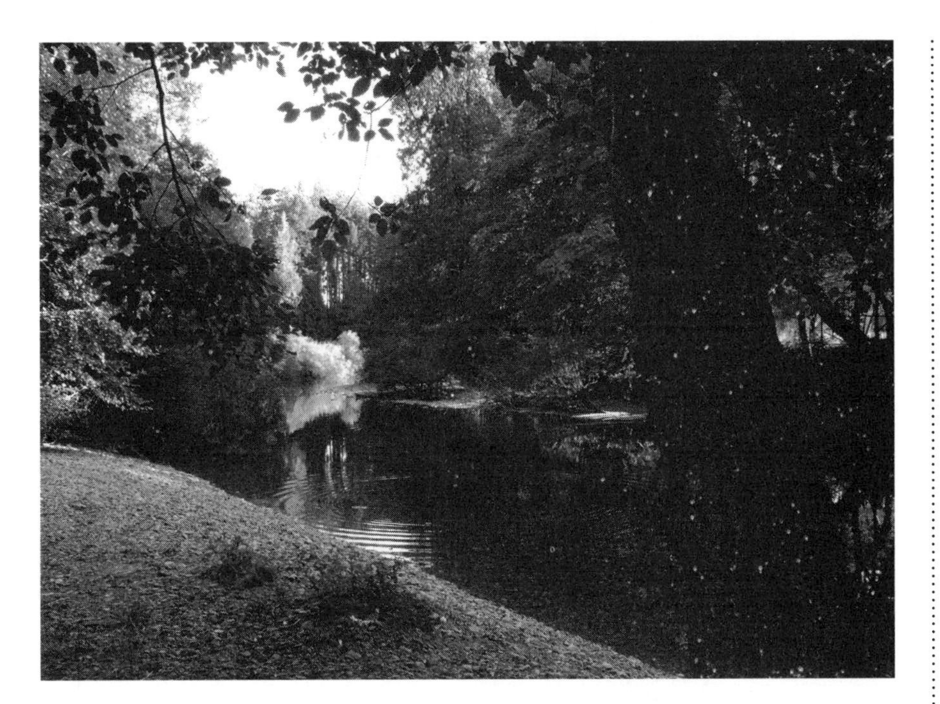

What animals eat, move, think, and interact in significantly different ways than their ancestors?

I am fortunate enough to own some property on a salmon river (pictured above). Every year when the salmon come to spawn and the bears and eagles come to feed, I am filled with a sense of gratitude and awe. I always think about how the DNA in the fish and eagles has been passed down from the ancestors of these animals for centuries and centuries. I think about how these animals, like all animals on earth except humans, are eating, moving, thinking and interacting as their ancestors did. I think about the wisdom, not just the innate genetic intelligence, but the acquired lifestyle wisdom that is responsible for this pattern. I admire these animals, I am envious of them and I am also apologetic and often ashamed of many of the actions of my species.

The fact is that for the vast majority of time that humans have been on earth we have been wild animals living amongst other wild animals in natural environments. It is only recently that we have become wild animals living in captivity in artificial environments away from wild animals. Since we have made this change, our health, and the health of the planet, has been in steady decline.

One of the most shocking things for me was when I was about 16 years old I read that one of the most dangerous things threatening the survival of the Fraser River salmon stocks was the sewage being pumped into the river. It was not the urine and the feces of humans, it was the pharmaceutical drugs and other chemical toxins found

> "By that time (1970s) industry had produced – and stashed SOMEWHERE – about 100 trillion pounds of hazardous wastes, enough wastes to create a highway to the moon 100 feet wide, 10 feet deep."
>
> Davis, Devra. The Secret History of the War on Cancer. 2007. Basic Books, a division of the Perseus Books Group. New York. NY.

in the feces and urine and all the chemicals from detergents and fertilizers and pesticides. This discovery still affects me. It was then that I started reading and learning about all the other pollutants that we were dumping into the environment. I had a moment in my life when I said, you know, there's nothing I can do for the wild animals unless I change the beliefs and behaviors of the domesticated human animals. You see, the truth is that we get to choose whether or not all the animals survive, we will ultimately determine if life on earth survives, at least as we currently know it. I don't say these things to convince you to eat granola and hug trees. I say these things so that you can realize that humans can only be healthy if we have a healthy ecosystem on the planet. If what we do kills other animals what do we think it is going to do to us?

If how we live causes other species to get sick and go extinct, can we remain unaffected?

I came to realize that the reason these wild animals were getting sick was because we were destroying their environments.

Around the same time, I concluded that the reason animals in captivity are obese and do not reproduce well, if at all, display aggressive and depressive behavior, and are generally much sicker and less vibrant than their genetically identical, wild cousins, is not due to their genes, but due to their wild genes being exposed to captive environments.

Remember these concepts, they are very important.

Accurately Defining Health and Sickness

Before we can have a meaningful discussion about health and sickness we need to understand what health and sickness represent. In science we would say that we need to operationally define our terms. Most people don't know the true meanings of health and sickness. Most doctors don't. Most nurses don't. Most teachers don't. Most parents don't. Most industrialized humans don't. A majority of industrialized humans are sick and will remain sick until they gain this understanding.

Developing your understanding of what health and sickness really represent is the foundation of what is required for you to be empowered to take control of your own health destiny; it is the foundation of living a better, longer life.

I distinctly remember one of the great moments of awareness and understanding I had about the true nature of health and sickness. I remember deeply contemplating the issue of endangered or extinct animal species. I thought to myself, of all the species that have ever gotten sick, become endangered, or gone extinct, none have ever been found to have done so because of genes. Think about that for a second. Of all of the species on the planet, there hasn't been a single case of a species getting sick, quite rapidly over 20, 30, 40, 50, or 100 years, where biologists or anyone else has blamed genes. Not a single case.

Of all the species that have ever gotten sick, become endangered, or gone extinct, have any done so because of bad genes?

Now put that in context with the fact that human chronic illness rates are rising rapidly. Since 1980, there has been a rapid increase in the per person rate of chronic illness in the United States and every industrial society. Chronic illness rates are rising even more rapidly in developing nations. Let's look at the per capita chronic illness rates in the United States since 1980. Over 46 percent of the United States population – that is mirrored exactly in Canada, and virtually every other Industrial nation by the way – currently has a chronic illness. This accounts for 78 percent of

"Not surprisingly, chronic diseases have become the leading cause of death and disability in the United States."

"Seven out of every 10 deaths are attributable to chronic disease, and illnesses like heart disease and cancer top the list of most common causes of death."

Almanac of Chronic Disease, 2009 Partnership to Fight Chronic Disease all healthcare spending.[8] The number of prescriptions per person is doubling every decade. Seventy-six percent of Americans regularly take prescription drugs.[9] Americans consume 25 million pills per hour every day yet millions still die every year of chronic illness.[10] Blaming genes and consuming pills are just not logical, scientific, or evidence-based approaches for wellness and prevention.

My next big "Ah Ha" moment was when I realized that humans were animals. The thing that allows you to feed your children things that you wouldn't feed your dog, the thing that allows you to say I just have to get my dog out for a walk and then leave your kid on the couch playing video games, the thing that allows you to choose these behaviors without any conscious concern is the belief system that you are not an animal.

You think humans are somehow physiologically different from animals, you think the natural laws that govern animals don't apply to humans. You're wrong – DEAD WRONG.

Are humans an animal species?

Rainforest Analogy

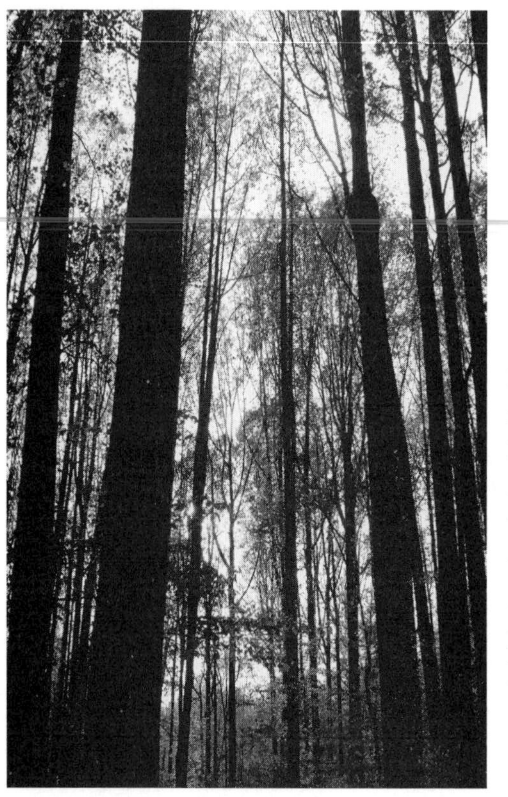

Let's begin to discuss the concept of health in more detail. The first thing I need you to realize if you are going to understand the true nature of health and sickness is that you are an ecosystem of cells. Consider a rainforest. A rain forest is made up of individual trees and the health of the rainforest, as a whole, is based upon the collective health of the individual trees. Thus as goes the health of the individual trees, so goes the health of the rain forest.

You, as a multicellular organism, are made up of an ecosystem of individual cells. So, like the rainforest, your health, as a whole ecosystem, is based upon the collective health of your individual cells. As goes the health of your individual cells, so goes the health of your whole ecosystem. If all of your cells are healthy, you are expressing your health potential. If some of your cells are sick, you are sick and you are not expressing your health potential.

Humans have about 75 trillion genetically identical cells that make up our bodies and brains (our ecosystem). Think about this fact while you are reading later chapters regarding the distinction between genetic expression and genetic code. Think about how different your eye cells are from your liver cells from your intestinal cells from your gonadal cells from your hair cells. All these different types of cells in your body and brain, which have vastly different structure and function, are genetically identical. So what makes these cells have different structure and function is not their genes but how these genes are being expressed. Same genes – EXACTLY – with VASTLY DIFFERENT structure and function.

Are humans, or any other species, genetically programmed to express sickness and develop chronic illness?

Chronic illness is not due to the expression of pathological genes or genes that have evolved to produce cancer, diabetes, obesity or any other chronic disease. Humans, like every other species on earth, get chronic illness because they get chronically exposed to a pathological environment that causes the genetic expression of stressed or adaptive physiology. It's the environment that's either normal or pathological, not our genes.

Our genes are the constant in the health equation; it is the environment and the expression of our genes that are variable or plastic.

What cellular biologists like Dr. Bruce Lipton (you will learn more about him later) see at a cellular level when they change the health of stem cells by changing their environment in a petri dish is exactly what I see at a clinical level when I take patients out of their toxic environment and get them to eat, move and think differently. Humans are a collection of cells living in a giant petri dish. We are an ecosystem of cells living in a giant petri dish ecosystem called earth. Now whether you think evolution is responsible for the cells and petri dish or you think God is responsible for the cells and the petri dish is not relevant to these facts. Whether God or evolution is responsible for the laws of the universe and the laws of physiology one thing is clear. Humans are governed by these laws and we break them at our own peril.

Visual Analog Scale for Health

Let's get back to accurately defining health and sickness. In science we call the state of healthiest cell function homeostasis. What this refers to is cells that are free of stressors and able to expend their energy on metabolic activities for maintaining growth and repair. For the purpose of this discussion we can just refer to this as a state of balance and harmony or a state of healthy cell function. If all of your cells are in a state of health they are not under any form of chronic stress and they are free to express their potential for health and vitality. We will call that 10 out of 10 on the visual analog scale of health and function. If you have zero out of 10 then you would have no function in any of your cells; that represents death. Anywhere in between zero and 9.999 means you are expressing less than your genetic potential for health and vitality.

Is state of cell function constant or does it change? Are changes random or in response to need?

So if we are at 10 out of 10 on the scale, is it possible for us to be sick? No. It's not possible, because sickness, by definition, is a lack of health, a lack of homeostasis, a lack of balanced and harmonious cell function. Sickness is stressed cell function. What sickness really represents is your cells in a state of adaptive function. Your cells are adapting to some form of stressor. There are some important questions about this that warrant further consideration. First of all, is there anyone reading this who believes that your state of cell function is determined by random chance? I hope not because this could not be further from the truth. In fact, life itself could be defined as a lack of randomness. If our cells functioned randomly, we would be incapable of survival. Life is, by definition,

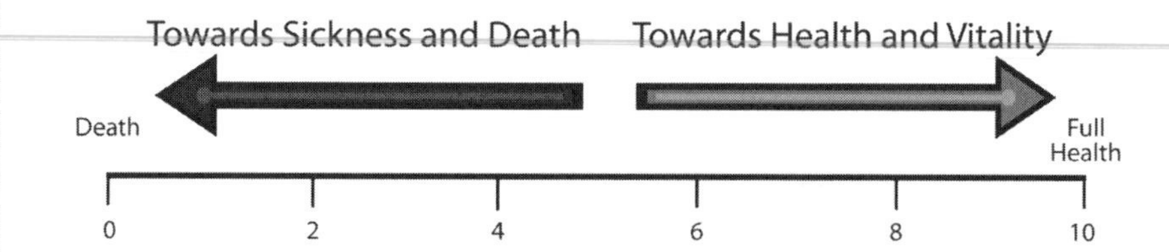

order rather than randomness, it is organization rather than entropy. So, our state of cell function is absolutely not determined by random chance.

Is there anyone who believes that humans, or any other species, are genetically programmed to be sick or to develop chronic illness? Evolutionists would certainly disagree with such a stance. Genes get stronger within a species with time not sicker, therefore blaming a rapid rise in chronic illness rates on genes is completely contrary to the theory of evolution. Creationists would certainly disagree with such a stance. Surely God did not create humans with flawed genes. Free will to make bad decisions, yes. Faulty genes, no. Chronic adaptive cell function, chronic stressed cell function, chronic illness, is definitely not caused by bad genes from either evolution or God.

The truth is that humans, like all living species, have cells that are genetically programmed to survive, to thrive, and to reproduce.

Do stressors come from inside genes, or do they come from the outside environment?

Because of our complexity and sheer number of cells, humans have developed a central nervous system to detect our environment and to control, regulate, and coordinate our cellular response to it. If I put you in the cold, you will shiver in order to raise your core temperature. If I cut your finger, your nervous system will send clotting and healing agents from your bloodstream to the site of injury. Really the definition of life is our ability to coordinate our ecosystem of cells to strive to survive and thrive. Our bodies do this constantly. We are in a world that has a lot of stressors in it, and what we are programmed to do is keep trying to get back to a state of balance.

The million dollar question is, "why would our cell function ever move away from a state of balance and toward a state of adaptive or stressed cell function?" It is not random chance. It is not because our cells are genetically programmed to move away from homeostasis, in fact, the exact opposite is true. Our cells are programmed to strive to survive and thrive, this is what keeps us alive. Why would we ever be in a state of sickness instead of a state of full health? The answer is stressors, some form of stressors.

I will define and describe stressors and their role in chronic illness in great detail in a later chapter but for now let me just give you a brief summary. A stressor must be defined in a species specific way, in a genetically specific way. Things that humans genetically require in terms of nutrition, or exercise, or energy expenditure, or socialization, may in fact be harmful or deadly to another species. It is our human genome that determines what is required to express our health potential, and it is our genome that determines what is stressful and causes us to express a state of adaptation or illness.

A stressor, most accurately defined, is a stimulus that elicits a state of adaptation, that elicits a move away from homeostasis and toward a state of adaptive physiology.

This brings us to yet another very important question. Do such stressors come from inside genes or from the outside environment?

The prevailing medical paradigm is that humans are sick with chronic illness because of problems that arise from within, from bad genes or bad cells. As widely held a belief as this is, it is inaccurate.

What is a stressor?

This paradigm is the source of so much of what is wrong with modern medical research and modern medical intervention. The failure of medicine to solve chronic illness is certainly not due to a lack of intelligent or, in my opinion, from a lack of caring practitioners. The failure is due to the wrong paradigm. The failure is due to the fact that allopathic or traditional medical research and intervention are conducted within the Sickness & Treatment Paradigm instead of the Wellness & Prevention Paradigm.

The reason humans, and every other species, move away from a state of health is because we are exposed to stressors that originate from the external, rather than internal, environment of our cells.

Let me ask you another important question. If I tell you that you are at 7 out of 10 on the health and cell function scale, are you sick? Yes, you are sick. Are you sicker if you are at 6 out of 10? Yes. Are you really sick if you are at 1 out of 10? Yes, really sick, almost dead.

If you are at 7 out of 10 on the health scale (expressing only 70 percent of your genetic potential for health) and we want to get you healthier, what is the only way that we can improve your health and well being? We are not going to change your genetic potential and why should we, your potential is fine. The fact that you are not expressing your potential cannot be blamed on your potential, that would be an absurd circular argument. If we want to get you, or any other human, or any member of any other species for that matter, healthier, we have to move cell function towards 10. We don't have to get all the way to 10 to realize significant health benefits. We have to get to 10 to reach our potential, but if you are sick and we want you to get healthier, all we have to do is move your cell function in the right direction. We have to move your cell function closer to homeostasis. Most importantly, we have to figure out what stressors are forcing your cells into a state of adaptation and take steps to remove these stressors. Do drugs and surgery move cell function towards 10?

As long as people can convince you that your physiology is somehow magical, and that you are not governed by the same natural laws as every other animal, then they can convince you that you can behave in ways that would make other animals sick while you somehow remain magically unaffected.

Why do people choose so many unhealthy behaviors?

If you believe this you can be convinced that it is safe to feed your kids soda and chips, but that these things would harm your dog and every other animal on earth. Sounds ridiculous when you actually read it put in those terms doesn't it?

The real insidious threat is that as long as you believe this, you will also freely believe that you don't have any power or responsibility when it comes to determining your own health.

You can be easily convinced that what you choose has little influence on your health and that whether or not you get sick or stay well is based on which genes you inherit and which drugs and surgery you have access to. In this paradigm you really have no power because your decisions don't really matter.

The reason why you regularly engage in unhealthy behaviors, and the reason why you both role model and abet your children to do the same, is because deep down you don't really feel like it matters that much. It is not because you are lazy, it is not because you are unintelligent, and it is not because you don't care.

Those choices don't matter that much to you because you have a belief system that says they don't matter in terms of your health and your quality and quantity of life. Think about it. If I put arsenic in the junk food you wouldn't feed it to yourself or your kids. Why not? Because the amount that such a choice mattered to you would be exponentially increased. All the reasons why you chose that food in the past would remain the same; what would change are the reasons you now had for not choosing that food. The same is true for those things you currently do not choose that you should. It's all about what matters to us.

Changing your behaviors is really about changing your belief systems, because it is your belief systems that determine what and how much things matter to you and our behaviors are based on what matters to us.

Would you eat your favorite junk-food or feed it to your children if you knew it had been laced with arsenic?

You don't equate poor eating, moving, and thinking choices with early death, cancer, diabetes, heart disease, ADHD, acne, acid reflux, depression, anxiety, Alzheimer's, and dementia. You don't equate poor food choices or sedentary patterns or negative thoughts, emotions and relationships with chronic illness and early death. As importantly, you also don't equate healthy food choices or regular exercise patterns or positive thoughts, emotions and relationships with significantly reduced risk of chronic illness or with a happier, longer, and better life. *Not yet. Not yet you don't.* Your beliefs and your life are about to change.

Chapter 2
Humans: Wild Animals in Captivity

"We habitually think or speak of ourselves as something apart from Nature, as belonging to some higher order of reality, when, in fact, we are as much a part of the total scheme of things as are the trees and the beasts of the field."

John Burroughs

"The city is not a concrete jungle. It is a human zoo."

Desmond Morris

Are humans governed by the same biological laws that govern every other animal species?

I believe the only way you are going to really understand the truth about health and sickness, take these truths to heart, and act upon them, is by understanding that your physiology is governed by the same biological laws as every other animal.

You must understand that humans are an animal species, a species of mammal with mammalian requirements for health.

I don't know where the false idea and belief system that humans are not an animal species or governed by the same natural laws that govern all other animal species came from. Maybe from health science, if so it was bad science. Maybe from religious teachings, if so they were they were false or misinterpreted religious teachings. I think that a fair assessment would put equal blame on both faulty science and faulty religious teachings, but I don't really care about blame. I only care about solutions.

Whatever the cause, I can tell you that it is quite clear now that we have totally lost the concept that we are part of the animal kingdom. I don't care how much or little you know about science or what your religious beliefs are because neither can change the fact that humans are an animal species and the natural laws that govern us are the same that govern all other animals species.

The source of these laws (God, Mother Nature, or both) is

irrelevant to the fact that these natural laws exist and govern us. People with all different science backgrounds, and all different religious beliefs, are dying by the millions because of how they eat, move, and think. Clearly these natural laws do not discriminate. What will happen to these poor people after they die I don't know, I won't even pretend to have any expert opinion in this area. However, the fact that they are dead and that they are dead early, too early, and that they are dead because their physiology was adversely affected by poor lifestyle choice is indisputable. I have a lot of expert opinion to share in this area.

Let's expand this idea a little further, let's start to ask questions that are based upon seeing humans as an animal species within this lifestyle-centric, naturalist paradigm. How many of you can drink the water from a stream within five miles of your house?

I live in Victoria, British Columbia, Canada. We have some of the cleanest and purest land, air, and water in North America. However, I will tell you that there are probably very few, if any, people in my area that can safely drink water from a stream within five miles of their house. What about where you live? Was this true 300 years ago? Of course not, everybody got water from a source near where they lived.

Can you safely drink the water from the streams within a five mile radius of your house?

Now I'm usually lecturing in large cities like New York or Chicago or Dallas or Toronto or London or Edinburgh or Sydney or Melbourne. Imagine drinking water from a stream within five miles of any of these cities! How can we believe that we can poison our streams and not poison ourselves?

How can we think that the animals are dying in these streams, and that somehow, magically, we will remain unaffected? This view makes no sense if you understand biological ecosystems.

How many of you would like to drink the water from the runoff of the farm that grows your childrens' fruit and vegetables? Now, does it make any sense that this doesn't concern us? I travel to Australia to lecture three or four times a year. That's a 15 hour flight at about 600 miles an hour, over the Pacific Ocean. It's water the whole time, it's a big ocean. For the entire flight there's not a spot in that ocean where we can't detect PCBs or fire retardant. We only

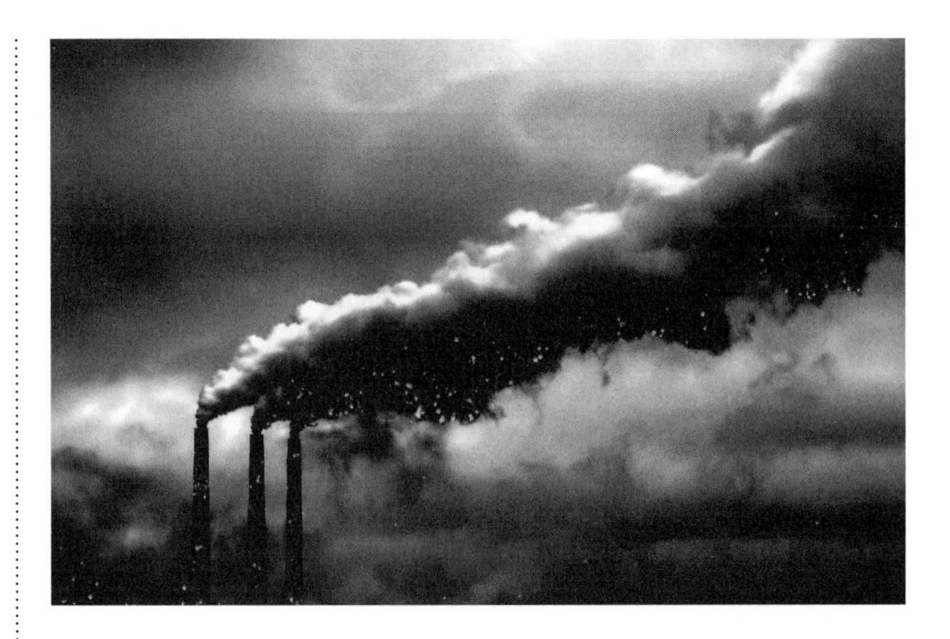

started using these chemicals a few decades ago. The solution to pollution is not dilution. We have soiled our own home – the earth.

Is it possible to pollute the water and soil and not ourselves?

The Orca whales living in the Strait of Juan de Fuca are now so toxic with fire retardant, PCBs, and DDT, that biologists fear for their survival. A study recently conducted in Washington State found over 200 industrial chemicals in the maternal blood of pregnant humans.[11] Many of these chemicals were known to be toxic, but most disturbingly, most have never even been tested. There are virtually no laws that require chemical companies to prove that their products are safe for the environment, for humans, or for other animals.

"Researchers at several nearby universities recently examined the genes of people who have been catching and eating fish heavily contaminated with DDT for nearly fifty years. Those who had eaten the most fish had the greatest numbers of abnormal cells and risk of breast cancer."

Davis, Devra. The Secret History of the War on Cancer. 2007. Basic Books, a division of the Perseus Books Group. New York. NY.

Now the point of this book is not to get all environmental and I don't want any political opinions or economic viewpoints to get in the way of facts, so let's just stick with what is indisputable. The truth is that the environment will never be a priority until you understand that you are part of it and that it is the source of your life. Again, in terms of relevance to this issue, it does not matter if you are going to heaven or not after there is no longer life on earth. What matters for this discussion is the unequivocal, indisputable fact that life on earth is a product of the resources from the earth.

Who or what created the earth is, once again, not relevant to this issue so please don't let it cloud your thinking. Regardless of your view on the issue of whom or what created the earth, or what will happen to you when it can no longer sustain life, the one thing that is indisputable is that the earth is the source of physical life while we are living upon it.

I really don't think we're going to be able to understand and own this concept until we understand who we really are. We are earth. We are animated earth. There is nothing in you that is not earth. You cannot pollute the earth without polluting me and my family, and I can't pollute the earth without polluting you and your family. We live on a recycling depot. Humans are an ecosystem of cells that live in ecosystems on a planet, which is an ecosystem in a universe, which is in an ecosystem of its own.

Are the earth's resources for life constantly replenished or just recycled and reused?

We live on a recycling depot. We literally drink dinosaur tears. The truth is that we ingest or absorb all the wastes, flesh, garbage, and chemicals that our ancestors have deposited into the earth.

I'm not convinced that global warming is really our biggest issue. I'm not sure that global warming is not turning into a giant diversion from the real issue. Let me ask you this question. Do we really care what temperature the earth is if it is so toxic that we can't inhabit it or eat or drink from it? Do we really care if it is one degree warmer or two degrees colder if it's so polluted that we can't eat anything that grows from it, or breathe the air that surrounds it? I'm not sure that temperature is the big issue, folks. The big issue is the cause of our sick planet and the sick inhabitants of our planet. Global warming is an effect, whether caused by normal cycles, by humans, or by a combination of both, it is not the main issue.

I completed 14 years of post-secondary education. One of the degrees I earned is a Master's Degree in science, human physiology to be specific. One of the things that always seemed so incongruent to me was that I could study the physiology of every species from a frog to a chimpanzee in the same biology class but if I wanted to study human physiology I had to go, not only to a different classroom, but outside of the biological department altogether. I had to leave and go to a different building to study human physiology. Why?

We have restaurants now that display signs reading, "no animals allowed," and they are full of people eating.

Stop and think for a moment about how often you refer to every species of animal under one heading and then speak about or refer to yourself or other people as humans, but not animals. This is important; this false belief has shaped not only our thoughts and behaviors but also our education and healthcare systems.

Why do we study animals separately from humans? What is this separation based on?

When I first had the realization that humans had become the sickest species on the planet, I really started researching to find out why this had occurred. I couldn't find a single documented example of an animal species that had gotten sick, become endangered, or gone extinct because of genes. In every case it was the environment. In fact, the theory of evolution itself is based on the idea that genes get better over time, that organisms get better adapted to their environments over time. Blaming genes for sickness goes against the theory of evolution and this is, of course, why biologists never blame genes for the sicknesses and extinction of animal species. In fact when I looked at the modern animal species that were sick, or endangered, or had recently gone extinct, what I found was that, in virtually every case, it had been humans that had caused the environmental change that was responsible. I remember discussing this with my father, a Ph.D. biologist. I asked him if he could think of any exceptions to this conclusion - he couldn't.

I also started to think about the fact that animals in captivity so often become sick, overweight, have fertility issues, become aggressive with each other, and die early. I asked myself, if we take a chimpanzee, the animal most genetically similar to humans, out of the wild and we put that chimpanzee into an environment that essentially makes it live like a human, does that chimpanzee get sicker or healthier? Sicker. How many times out of a million? A million times out of a million.

I realized that, as simple as this concept was, it was very significant. I then asked the next logical question. If I wanted to get these sick chimpanzees in captivity well, what would I need to do? What questions would I need to ask? Should I ask how to diagnose or label the sicknesses of those chimpanzees and ask which drugs to give them to treat the symptoms? Should I figure out which body parts I could remove or bypass? Should I create a whole system based on labeling those states of sickness of those chimpanzees in captivity so that I could sell drugs to all the zoo keepers and veterinarians? Should I then blame these sicknesses on genes and thus remove any responsibility to create a healthy environment for these animals in captivity and make everyone believe such illnesses were inevitable or caused by old age? Should I also create an insurance industry to make money from these sick animals? Should I create a pharmaceutical industry to make money from these sick animals? I guess it depends on whether my motivation was to make money or to get the sick animals well.

If animals put into captivity get sick would it be logical to blame genes?

Or, should I ask why these chimpanzees are sick. Should I ask what makes these sick chimpanzees different from the healthy ones and try to isolate these factors so I can address them? Now, in biology, that makes total sense. As a trained biologist, that's the first thing that you would ask.

As a biologist, if you observed an animal species becoming sick or dying off, you would never assume the issue was genes; that would simply be ludicrous.

The first thing you would do is figure out what was going on in the environment of that animal that is making it sick. Isn't that logical? Of course it is. So that's what I did. I studied the healthy animals in the wild, and I compared them to the sick animals in captivity and the first thing I learned was that there was no difference in their genes – none. The second thing I learned is that we could always attribute their illnesses to their lifestyle changes, to the changes in their environment. To be specific, to the changes in their lifestyle that represented moving away from what was genetically congruent for that species toward what was genetically incongruent. From an environment that supplied the genetically required raw materials and avoided toxicity to an environment that failed to supply genetically required raw materials and exposed them to many toxins.

At this point, I started to realize that it would be absurd beyond belief to think that the way to get sick chimpanzees well would be to add drugs or take away body parts. The only thing that made sense was to realize that, if I wanted healthy chimpanzees in captivity, they would require an environment that mimics the one that the healthy chimpanzees enjoy in the wild. The sick chimpanzees in captivity would need to eat, move and think like the healthy chimpanzees in the wild. It makes perfect sense doesn't it? It is so logical that it is almost to the point that it seems too obvious. It is obvious, it is really self evident – IF you ask the right questions.

Great Lakes Analogy

What is the difference between healthy wild animals and sick animals in captivity? What is making the animals in captivity sick?

Allow me to use an analogy to help you ask the right questions. I find that most people have been so indoctrinated into the current paradigm that they simply filter out a lot of what they see, hear, and read. I will use a lot of analogies and a lot of the Socratic method to get you to THINK and to get you to see the world through a different lens, within a different paradigm. You will learn, and experience, that changing your paradigm can change your conclusions, even though you are presented with the same information.

Do you remember when, or are you at least aware of the fact that, the fish in the North American Great Lakes started dying and washing up on shore in large numbers during the 1970s? They started washing up on the shore with tumors. The same thing is happening to the Beluga whales in the St. Lawrence today and to other species all over the world that are being exposed to industrial toxins. Do you also remember or are you aware of what happened to the birds that ate those fish? Their eggs became brittle and they were not producing offspring, and scientists and environmentalists were very worried about the extinction of the birds, as well as the fish.

How many of you think any biologist or any other kind of scientist in their right mind would have come to the conclusion that the problem with the fish in the Great Lakes was due to their genes? How many of you believe that scientists concluded that the reason those fish developed cancer, or whatever other illnesses they

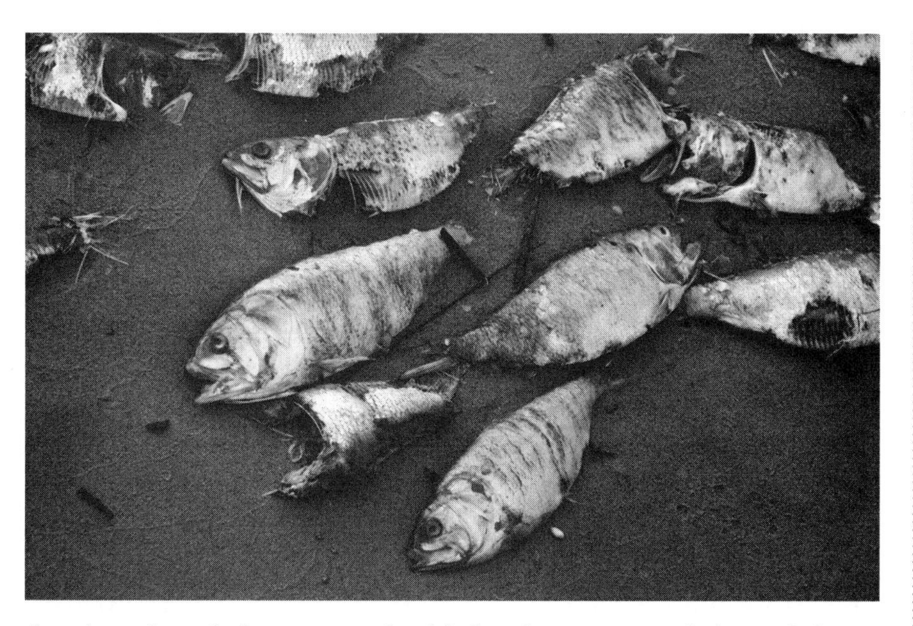

developed, and the reason the birds who consumed those fish got so sick, was due to bad genes? How many of you think that any biologist came to the conclusion that a logical solution was to dump chemotherapy and other drugs into the lakes, or set up little, tiny, fish and bird hospitals with little, tiny, fish and bird instruments on the shores of the lakes, so that when the sick birds and fish washed up they could give them drugs, radiation and surgery?

In the 1970's, when the birds and fish in the great lakes started getting sick and dying, did any biologist blame genes?

How many of you think that would be logical? I'm sure none of you. Now I need to ask you a very important, very paradigm shifting question. Why would you think such an explanation or approach is logical for the human species? Why would it be viewed as absurd to suggest this approach for any other animal species on earth yet seen as virtually blasphemous to suggest any other approach for the human animal species? There are several reasons for this and once I can get you to understand the source of such an illogical belief system I can get you to easily discard it.

One reason is because it is very uncomfortable to talk about human sickness. Sickness is a human tragedy and it is very difficult to discuss personal responsibility because many people mistake this for blame. It is not blame, it is empowerment to help prevent future illness and to recover from present illness. I still find this uncomfortable to do at times. However, if I don't do it, it is more uncomfortable.

If I don't tell the truth and I let people continue to commit suicide with their choices because I was too uncomfortable to tell the truth, then everyone I didn't tell the truth to haunts me. I've murdered those people with an act of omission. I am determined and devoted to tell you the truth, and I will also tell you that I have the data to support what I will tell you. I am going to show you that data in this book and, although at first it may terrify you or anger you, it will eventually inspire you and empower you. The truth, as always, can set you free.

However, until you understand the truth it may indeed be an uncomfortable time for both of us. A lot of you are going to go through some uncomfortable moments as you read this book. A lot of you are going to find out that you could have done a better job in terms of your own health, and you could have done a better job for the health of your children. What I want to tell you is that the choices you made in the past were based on the belief systems you had in the past. You can't change the past. Guilt can't serve you, so don't choose that path.

If we do not know the truth about our own responsibility regarding our health and illness, how can we ever recover from illness, or prevent ourselves or others from getting sick?

I respect you too much to avoid telling you the truth based on the arrogant and disempowering assumption that you cannot handle it or would rather not hear it. Avoiding telling you the truth prevents you from helping yourself or the ones you love. It is neither ethical nor moral.

I am not suggesting it is your fault if you are sick, I am suggesting, in fact I am insisting, that your choices are the most important thing determining your health and recovery and it is imperative that you fully understand the consequences of your choices. Ignorance is not bliss. Ignorance costs lives - millions and millions of lives.

We have created this artificial division between our physiology and how our bodies function and how the bodies of the rest of the species on the planet function. This belief system has allowed us, or perhaps inevitably driven us, to become completely illogical and unscientific about the consequences of our choices and the treatments we provide. This belief system allows us to ignore our innate common sense, it allows us to be convinced that we need experts in sickness in order to be healthy. It has caused us to become the sickest species on the planet with the sickest offspring on the planet. It has caused us to be indifferent about causing the entire ecosystem of the earth to become sick. It allows us to do things that we know make other animals sick and extinct while we remain convinced that we can remain unaffected. It has allowed us to blame our exponentially rising rates of chronic illness, not on our behaviors or on the environmental changes we have caused, but on our genes, even though this is completely contrary to the gene theory itself and to what we conclude about every other animal species on the planet. It has allowed suicide by lifestyle choice to become the leading cause of death while drugs and surgery to treat the effects of this lifestyle have become the leading industry on the planet and the single greatest cause of government and corporate spending, debt, and bankruptcy.

Only when we are able to step back and see ourselves through the eyes of a biologist or a zoologist, rather than a pathologist or pharmacologist, will we grasp how and why humans have become the sickest species on earth and what humans need to do to get and stay well.

Is it possible to solve a problem if you have not correctly identified the cause? Why have humans become the sickest species on the planet?

There is no other mammalian species that comes close to the human species in terms of heart disease, cancer, obesity, diabetes, acid reflux, anxiety, depression, infertility, anger, murder, resentment, and lack of community.

We are in real trouble and until we understand why we are in trouble, our attempts to try to resolve our problems will not be effective. You cannot solve a problem until you identify and address the cause. In order to get the right answers, you must first ask the right questions. We have been asking the wrong questions. We have been asking how to diagnose and treat chronic disease and we have assumed that these diseases were genetic and thus inevitable and incurable. We were wrong.

The reason that I have been so successful in helping people get and stay well is because I have asked the right questions. The reason I have asked the right questions is because I have had the right paradigm. I have studied humans as an animal species.

I have started with the major premise that humans, like all other animal species, don't get sick because of genes but rather because of environment. For over 25 years I have used this major premise to form the right questions to find answers to why humans have become so sick and what we need to do to get and stay well.

As self-evident as these questions may appear to you, I am telling you that current health care curricula, research agendas, and practice guidelines are not focused upon asking and answering these questions. I can also tell you that this is precisely why we have a pandemic of chronic illness in the midst of a society that spends trillions of dollars on sickness care.

The current medical system is not failing because medical doctors are greedy, stupid, or indifferent. The system is failing because it is based on a paradigm that fails to study and care for humans as animals and has a belief system that blames genes rather than the environment for chronic illness. They believe illness is genetically predetermined, that illness is based on the inherent weakness of the organism rather than a genetically incongruent or toxic and deficient environment.

Does the current healthcare system view humans as an animal species?

The first thing we have to do is realize and accept the FACT that humans are an animal species, we have to accept the FACT that humans are wild animals living in captivity.

When we accept the FACT that humans are animals we will accept that if we want valid answers about the health of the human animal we are going to have to ask biological questions about the human animal; we are going to have to discover the natural environment, the genetically congruent environment, for the human animal species.

This is a profound paradigm shift from almost everyone else who is studying humans and this has made my research more difficult. It has been very challenging to sift through the tens of thousands of research articles to find a biological perspective on human health. The biological perspective has simply not been what has driven medical research or medical clinical interventions.

As I reviewed the literature over the past 25 years what became obvious to me was that, as long as medical research ignored the importance of environment and stayed focused on genes, they were never going to realize the true cause of illness or the true source of health and prevention.

As long as illness is viewed as being caused by genes or inherently weak cells, prevention and cure will never be seen as logical or possible clinical outcome goals. Instead, drugs to palliate what is seen as inevitable, incurable illness will continue to be the focus. The fact that drugs can neither prevent nor cure chronic illness will simply continue to be ignored as our attention continues to be focused on sickness and treatment instead of wellness and prevention. We will just continue down the road of more drugs and less health.

Truthfully, you could take the healthiest people in the world and give them prescription drugs, and they would always get sicker. Drugs don't make you healthy, they treat the effects of sickness. Healthy people are not supposed to take drugs – why? Because drugs make healthy people sick. Just think about that for a minute. This does not mean drugs are never appropriate, it means drugs never make you well.

If you took an aboriginal human being that lived as a hunter-gatherer and made her/him eat, move, think, and interact like the average industrial human would she/he get healthier or sicker?

Drugs can kill some pathogens and drugs can elicit changes in biochemistry but drugs cannot make you healthy. Only healthy living can make you healthy.

If we took a healthy human being, for example a healthy hunter-gatherer, and we made them eat, move, think, and interact like people in industrial society they would immediately get sicker. However, their genes would not change. You don't have to be a statistician or a Ph.D. mathematician to understand that if one variable like illness is rising and the other variable, genes, is not changing at all, you cannot logically attribute the cause of the rise in one variable to the variable that has remained unchanged.

There are some fundamentally important questions that arise within the biological perspective that is the foundation of the Wellness & Prevention Paradigm. Some of the most important questions I had to find answers to were, "what does the physiology of a healthy human being look like and how do healthy human beings eat, move, think, and interact?" "Are there any healthy human beings, are there any human beings living in a healthy environment?" I needed a gold standard for human health. I needed some healthy humans to use as a reference point. I needed an example that I could point to and say, "if you want to get and stay well, you need to eat, move, think, and interact like those healthy human animals."

I'm suggesting, in fact, insisting, that if we want to be healthy we need to mimic, as closely as possible, the eating, moving, thinking, and interacting patterns of healthy human beings. Success leaves clues, and of course, so does failure.

It took a lot of painstaking research and a lot of sorting through false claims – mostly by those trying to sell some secret health formula, supplement, or regime, but I did find a credible and validated population of healthy human subjects. They are called hunter-gatherers. Hunter-gatherers are wild human beings living outside of captivity. Hunter-gatherers are human animals living a genetically congruent lifestyle in genetically congruent environments. Don't panic, I'm not suggesting we all leave our homes and move into the forest or onto the savannah.

What is more genetically congruent for the human species, the hunter-gatherer or the industrial lifestyle? Which lifestyle would cause more chronic illness and which would result in greater health?

How many of you have seen that ridiculous picture where there is a bunch of dogs sitting around a table smoking cigars and playing cards? You probably got a giggle. Well, based on our physiology and what makes us sick or well, it is no more ridiculous, and no more genetically incongruent or unnatural, for the dogs to behave this way than for humans. You smoking a cigar, living an artificial life in toxin-filled buildings, consuming alcohol, potato chips and other toxins, playing cards and being sedentary, is no less absurd for you than it is for the dogs. This is the point that gets missed if we don't view humans as animals, we miss the fact that the consequences to those dogs for living that way are no different than the consequences for humans living that way. This very important point is being missed by those in charge of the entire health care system.

Humans don't have any magic genes or magic physiology that allows us to make consequence-free choices. We are not capable of living outside the biological laws of the universe. Genetically incongruent lifestyle choices affect us just like they affect all the other animals on earth.

So when I looked at these hunter-gatherers what I realized

was, that when we study hunter-gatherers, we find healthy populations. Even the elderly hunter-gatherers rarely, if ever, suffer from chronic illness. Statistically, not as many hunter-gatherers reached old age – about 20 percent did, but the ones who did remained well. More importantly, these 20 percent did not represent genetically "advantaged" individuals. Those that died before reaching old age were not genetically "disadvantaged".

"About 20% of hunter-gatherers reach age 60 or beyond but even in this age bracket, individuals from foraging and other technologically primitive cultures appear almost completely free from manifestations of most chronic degenerative diseases (osteoarthritis is an exception)."

Eaton SB, & Cordain L. Evolutionary health promotion: a consideration of common counterarguments. Prev Med 2002; 34:119-123.

Hunter-gatherers do not die young or old from chronic illness. They die from trauma, infection from trauma, or from starvation. Regardless of what they die from, hunter-gatherers live their lives free of chronic illness, they are healthy and fit and full of vitality. Hunter-gatherers live better lives, shorter or longer, and the variable determining whether they live as long as industrial human beings has nothing to do with their genes or their access to drugs and surgery for chronic illness.

Why did the elderly in hunter-gatherer populations remain virtually free of chronic illness?

Think of the natives who lived where you live before industrialized, domesticated, white man showed up. I call this race of humans Whitey. Whitey showed up with what? White bread, white flour, white sugar, white milk, and white doctors in white coats prescribing white pills. The Whitey Plague, as I like to call it.

Whitey said don't eat that fresh fish and wild game meat or those fresh berries, or fresh tubers because that's uncivilized, it is barbaric. You need civilized Whitey food. When those native hunter-gatherers started eating this Whitey food, how did that go for them? Did they get sicker or healthier? They got sicker, a lot sicker.

Was it their genes? Of course not. Ironically, we actually have people now arguing that because native populations living the Whitey lifestyle in Whitey industrialized society have such high chronic illness rates (more obesity, diabetes, etc) that they must somehow be genetically weak or genetically predisposed to chronic illness.

They are now making the case that chronic illness itself must be a genetic problem. But how can it be genetic? For thousands of generations there was NO OBESITY OR DIABETES in these populations. When Whitey showed up with the Whitey Plague these populations developed these problems within one generation. How can it be genes?

Chapter 3
Paradigm and Research: The Question is Everything

"The scientist is not a person who gives the right answers, he's the one who asks the right questions."

Claude Levi-Strauss

"Sometimes the questions are complicated and the answers are simple."

Dr. Suess

Are the "healthy" subjects in medical research actually healthy?

One of the biggest weaknesses of Sickness & Treatment Paradigm research is how they define healthy subjects. They completely ignore the very important fact that they are studying wild, human animals in captivity. The subjects in their studies are living in genetically incongruent environments, are exposed to chronic stressors, and are thus either ill, or in a stage of developing illness. For this reason, it can appear, especially if you believe that genes determine health, that humans inevitably develop illness based on their genetic makeup. Make no mistake about it, this is the underlying belief system of traditional medicine and medical science when it comes to chronic illness.

If we look at what happens now, if we look at medical research, one of the most fundamental flaws with the validity of current medical research is how they define health and sickness.

Traditional medical researchers are studying wild, human animals in captivity but they never even consider the fact that the human in front of them is an animal in a captive, genetically incongruent, unhealthy environment. Traditional medical research will report that they compared healthy subjects to sick subjects or that they studied either healthy or sick subjects. But how do they define health and sickness? Do they define a healthy subject as somebody who lives the genetically congruent lifestyle for the human species? Do they define a healthy subject as someone who eats healthy foods, who is physically fit, who has a healthy body composition, who has a high level of self-esteem, a high level of life enjoyment, who has healthy social connections? No, they don't define health this way at all.

Traditional medical research most often defines a healthy subject as someone who has not been diagnosed with the illness or disease that is under investigation. So if the study is about heart disease anyone without a diagnosis of heart disease is defined as a healthy subject. Does being free of the diagnosis of heart disease actually mean they are healthy? Does it mean that they are not depressed? Does it mean that they can do five chin ups? Does it mean that they can jog two miles without stopping? Does it mean that they love themselves? Does it mean that they have positive self esteem? Does it mean that they eat good foods? No, it most certainly does not mean any of this.

We need to question the validity of this paradigm. We don't just need to question the methods and results, the drugs and the surgeries, the deaths and side effects, the lack of cures, the increasing incidence of illness, the escalating costs, the lack of scientific evidence. We need to question the paradigm that has created this approach and allows it to seem scientific and logical despite so much evidence to the contrary.

Is the lack of being diagnosed with a disease synonymous with being in good health?

This is really the fundamental difference between the Sickness & Treatment Paradigm and the Wellness & Prevention Paradigm. In the Sickness & Treatment Paradigm health has stopped being defined as a state of homeostasis, and has come to be defined as the absence of a diagnosed disease. Clearly the absence of a diagnosed disease is not an accurate definition of health.

The Plant Analogy

Let me give you an analogy to show you how important paradigm is in terms of health research and health care. Let's talk about plants. The reason I use plants will become obvious in a moment. Let me ask you a question. If you had a wilting plant what is the first thing you would do? I bet your answer was that you would either give it water or check the soil to see if it needed water. Why? Why didn't you answer that you would give it prescription drugs or check to see if it had enough prescription drugs? This is almost certainly what you would have answered if I had asked you

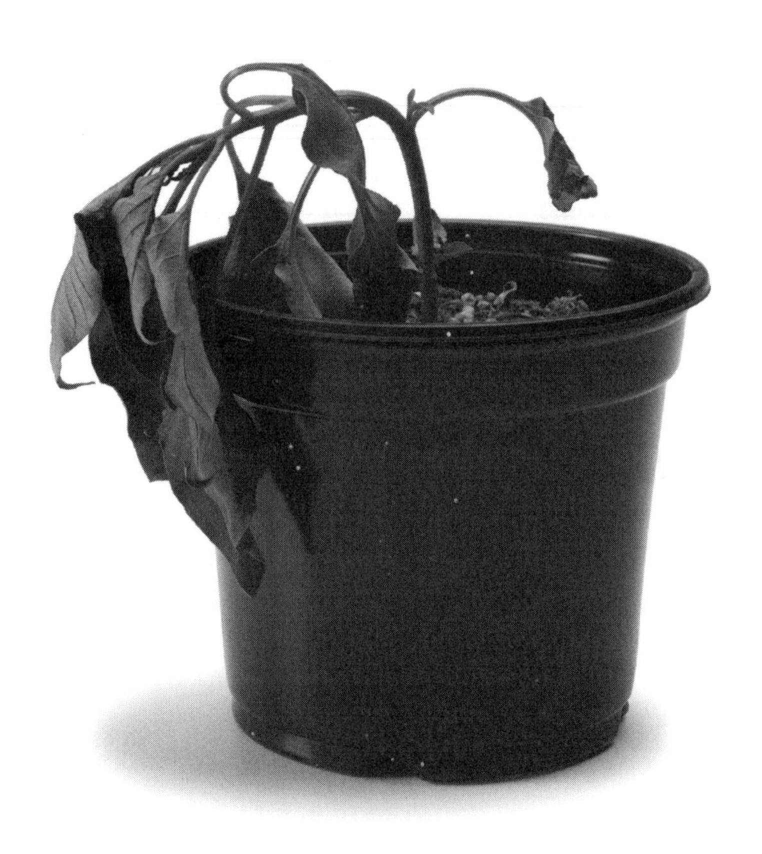

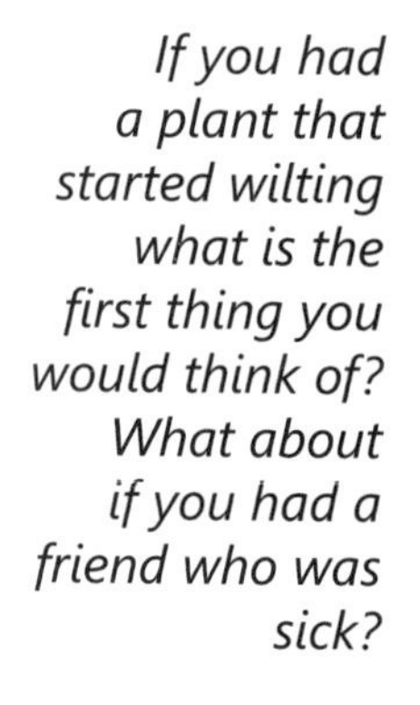

If you had a plant that started wilting what is the first thing you would think of? What about if you had a friend who was sick?

what you would do if you had a wilting or a sick human.

So why do most immediately think of a required nutrient for a plant but a drug for a human? The answer is because most view humans through a Sickness & Treatment Paradigm but all other living creatures through a Wellness & Prevention Paradigm. Their belief system is that the plant is genetically programmed to express health, that if the plant is wilting it must be toxic or deficient, probably deficient in water. Automatically when most think of nature, they presuppose that nature is programmed for survival and reproduction. That's the whole concept of Darwinian theory, that nature is programmed for success. Yet if I talk about humans, it's a completely different paradigm and belief system and thus a completely different set of questions, answers, and behaviors.

Let's get back to the plant. Imagine if you were a wilting plant in a study of many wilting plants. I'll be the researcher. The first thing I will need to do is randomly divide all of the wilting plants in the study into two groups. The gold standard in clinical research is a randomized, double blind, controlled trial. What does this mean? It means that we randomly assign each subject (in this example, each plant) in the study a number and then randomly assign each subject into a group. That is what randomized means. Controlled means that we are going to control all the other variables that could affect the results other than the one we're studying. This is really a fallacy if you are doing human studies because we cannot control the beliefs of a human being and the data is clear that the beliefs of a human being have a HUGE effect on results. So really controlled is misleading but that is a topic for another time.

Double blind means they poke out both eyes of the researcher. Not really, it's just a joke I can count on to get a laugh when I am lecturing to practitioners or students. Probably doesn't translate well to a book but I can't help myself. Double blind actually means that neither the researchers nor the subjects are aware of who is in what group. In other words neither the researchers nor the subjects know who is in the intervention group or the control group (the fake intervention group).

Do pharmaceutical companies conduct research to find out how to get sick people well or do they conduct research to find out how to get doctors to prescribe their drugs to sick people?

If you were a pharmaceutical company, what kind of double blind randomized controlled trials would you be conducting? What questions would you want the answers to? What questions would you pay money to get the answers to? You would pay money to find out whether or not your drug can have a desired effect and thus be sold for profit – BIG profit. What desired effect are they looking for? They are looking for a change in symptoms of course.

You have to understand that when people are studying how to treat symptoms and sickness, what they are really asking is whether or not they can make sick people feel better. They are not asking whether they can get sick people well.

This is not the question they are asking. They are asking if their drug can make sick people feel better, or whether it can change some of the physiological or biochemical variables or risk factors associated with disease. They are asking if they can make people appear less sick. How do they define sickness? They define sickness by symptoms or risk factors. It is really all about symptoms and nothing at all to do with health and function. It is completely symptom-centric.

Let me give you an example of both the lack of validity and the danger of this paradigm. Let's say that they divide all of the wilting plants into two equal groups. One group will receive real water and the other group will receive fake water or placebo water. At the end of six or eight or twelve weeks of the gold standard double blind trial, all of the plants are still wilting. What is the conclusion of the study? The conclusion of the study is that water is not a useful intervention for wilting plants. From this it could be, and often is, concluded that anyone who offers wilting plants water is not delivering evidence-based care and is thus either a fraud or a quack.

But you might say, "wait a minute, without water, plants will die." Sorry, that's not the question they asked; they did not ask if water was required by plants for survival or for health. They only asked whether or not giving water to wiling plants resulted in less symptoms, in less wilting to be precise. If the water did not result in less symptoms then water did not have a benefit - water did not result in the plants getting better, water was useless. Better is operationally defined by a decrease in symptoms, a decrease in wilting. Why do they get to define better as less wilting? Because that is how better is defined in the Sickness & Treatment Paradigm.

Does having less symptoms mean that you are healthier?

Now let's think about that for a second. What if I conducted the same study, used the same subjects, used the same intervention, got the same data, but I changed my question and my definition of better. What if I changed my question from a Sickness & Treatment Paradigm question to a Wellness & Prevention Paradigm question. What if I asked whether or not giving water to these plants could improve their cell function and health by moving them towards homeostasis?

Same data, same everything, the only thing I changed was the question. Really the only thing I changed was the paradigm of the researcher and as you will see this is EVERYTHING.

Now, the plants that were missing water, did they get better? Think about it for a second. Stop. I'll back up. Do plants need water? Obviously. These plants don't have enough. So I give them some. I give them the right amount. Did they get better? That depends how one defines "better," doesn't it? If you define better by symptoms, and they're still wilting or at least not wilting by a statistically significant less amount, then your conclusion would be that none of the plants got better. If you define better by moving towards homeostasis, and having better functioning cells, then any plant that got water got better - by deduction we know that cells that require water function better and are healthier when they have water. This creates a big difference, doesn't it? Our conclusion, with the same exact subjects, intervention, and data, goes from water is useless to water is a panacea!

You will come to understand that there are panaceas when it comes to wellness and prevention. Panaceas are simply those things that we genetically require to express health. If we need it, and are missing it, adding it represents a panacea. If it is toxic to us and we remove it, that represents a panacea.

If everyone is suffering from a deficiency of vitamin C or water, then vitamin C and water are panaceas for improving cell function in this population. Now imagine if, like me, you spent your life studying what the human species required in terms of raw materials from the environment in terms of eating, moving, thinking, and interacting. Imagine if you had unequivocal data from the most respected peer-reviewed journals in the world that substantiated the fact that the leading cause of death, suffering, bankruptcy, and the healthcare crisis was indeed deficiency in genetically required ingredients or raw materials and toxicity from genetically incongruent stressors.[12] Now imagine that the prevailing system was based not on supplying these sufficient materials or removing these toxins but rather on prescribing drugs to treat the symptoms of being deficient and toxic. *Welcome to my world.*

Is there such thing as a panacea for treating disease? Are there panaceas for creating better health?

What represents sufficiency in terms of the genetically required raw materials and what represents toxicity from genetically incongruent stressors is exactly what I have taught to over 5000 doctors in my wellness lifestyle certification program. The results have been extraordinary. I'll talk more about this in the final chapter.

We need to start asking ourselves how we should assess healthcare interventions. Should we assess interventions by whether or not they result in less symptoms or by whether or not they result in greater health? What makes more sense to you if you want to create a population that expresses more health and less illness? We are not asking these questions right now in traditional healthcare because traditional healthcare operates within the gene-centric Sickness & Treatment Paradigm. The results of this approach over the past 50 years have been well documented. The results have been devastating both in terms of health and expenditure.

Now you might logically ask, "if the plants are still wilting how can this Wellness & Prevention Paradigm model be worth anything? It may look good on paper but, in reality, would it not just result in a bunch of wilting plants with a little better function?"

Should we assess the value of a health care intervention based on whether it can help sick people feel better or whether it can get sick people well?

I hope you were asking that question because that is a great question. I LOVE good questions because good questions are the only way to find good answers. My first answer would be that just because the plants got water does not mean that we have solved all the issues of toxicity and/or deficiency. Perhaps the plants are also missing nutrients in their soil. The sobering reality of this is that if you were not asking what the plants were deficient in, if you were not operating within the Wellness & Prevention Paradigm, you would never ask these questions and you would never conduct these studies. Instead, you would just come up with a different drug to see if that drug could stop the wilting. If the leaves were brown, you would try and figure out something you could inject to make the leaves more green. You would never ask what was causing the problem. You would always ask what the treatment could be. This is a HUGE difference. The question is everything. If you do not ask the right question you will never get the right answer, regardless of how well designed the study is.

If you are operating within the paradigm or belief system that the cause of the problem was due to weak genes or weak cells you would not come up with the right questions. You would never ask what toxicity or deficiency caused the problem because you would be operating under the assumption that faulty genes or some inherent pathology was the cause of the problem. Nobody actually believes that humans are sick due to a deficiency of prescription drugs or that prescription drugs will restore health and function. Drug interventions are aimed at treating symptoms not at addressing causes.

Studies used as evidence for cholesterol and blood pressure drugs do not research the cause of high cholesterol or high blood pressure, they only study if the drugs they come up with can lower these risk factors. They also don't ask if lowering these risk factors increases health, the entire focus is on changing the risk factor. The problem is that the risk factor is an effect, it is not the cause of illness or a disease, it is simply one of the effects of being ill with a lifestyle caused illness. As Peter Sterling from the Department of Neuroscience, University of Pennsylvania points out, "Consequently despite the remarkable ingenuity, 30 years of low-level pharmacological treatments for hypertension have not worked. For the same reasons, it seems doubtful that low-level treatments for obesity and metabolic syndrome will be more successful, and already there have been serious adverse effects."[13]

"The inherent problem is that most pharmacologic strategies do not address the underlying causes of ill health in Western countries - which are not drug deficiencies."

Willet, W.C. (2002) Balancing Lifestyle and Genomics Research for Disease Prevention. Science 296: 695-698

Does evidence-based mean evidence for changing symptoms or evidence for improving health and function? What should it mean?

Let's get back to our research. Let's now give the plants water and nutrients. One of the groups of plants gets fake water and fake nutrients. Another group gets real nutrients and fake water. The third group gets real water and fake nutrients. The fourth group gets real water and real nutrients. Once again, at the end of the study, all of the plants are still wilting. Now, this is the gold standard, randomized double blind controlled trial. At the end of this gold standard study, all the plants are still wilting. What is the conclusion? The conclusion is that water and nutrients are no good for wilting plants. Anyone who offers or suggests offering water and nutrients for wilting plants would not be practicing evidence-based care and would be labeled a quack . But, wait, you might say, without water and nutrients, those plants will surely die. Sorry. That's not the question. In the gene-centric Sickness & Treatment Paradigm better is defined as less symptoms. This is especially true regarding drug research and the medical system is highly drug-centric.

The pharmaceutical companies that conduct the vast majority of clinical research and provide the vast majority of clinical education and send the pharmaceutical reps to visit every medical doctor's

> "In the U.S there are more drug industry lobbyists than members of congress."
>
> Katharine Greider. The Big Fix: How the Pharmaceutical Industry Rips Off American Consumers. 2003. Public Affairs.

office, and spend billions of dollars on political lobbyists and advertising campaigns are asking sickness and treatment not wellness and prevention questions.[14]

This paradigm and this way of thinking have dominated health care for a century, they have had trillions of dollars of government and private funding, they have had a carte blanche monopoly on healthcare and they have completely failed to prevent or solve the chronic illness pandemic.

If the only way to solve the chronic illness pandemic and the healthcare crisis is to have healthier people, and if drugs and surgery don't make people healthy, are more drugs and surgery scientific, logical or valid solutions?

The indisputable fact is that during this period, in the areas of the world that have spent the most money and have had the most access to sickness and treatment medical care, the citizens have gotten sicker and sicker every year. How can we even consider investing more money on this system or think that simply making this system more financially streamlined so we can apply it to more people who can't afford it is the solution? THIS IS INSANE!

Again, the ONLY solution to the chronic illness pandemic and the healthcare crisis it has caused, is to have FEWER SICK PEOPLE (or more people that are healthy). If people are sick because of lifestyle how on earth can we think that drugs and surgery are valid, logical, or scientific solutions for creating a society with fewer sick people?

Treating sickness will NEVER prevent sickness. Researching sickness treatments will NEVER produce useful information for wellness and prevention. It's not rocket science. It's just a simple matter of paradigm.

The only scientifically valid way to define health or better health is with respect to cell function. This is how physiologists define health. I have a Master's degree in physiological science and I can assure you that it is valid to define better in terms of whether or not cell function moves toward homeostasis. The truth is that you don't need a graduate degree in science to understand this; you just need some common sense. Let me ask you this question. If we know that plants need water and they need nutrients in the soil, and we give the plants the very water and nutrients they need, would they get better if we define better in terms of increased cell function rather than decreased symptoms? Of course they would.

> "To summarize, the body is actually a social order of about 100 trillion cells organized into different functional structures, each of which maintains homeostatic conditions in the internal environment. As long as normal conditions are maintained, the cells of the body continue to live and function properly."
>
> Guyton, Arthur C. Textbook of Medical Physiology, 8th edition. 1991. W.B. Saunders. Page 8.

Now I hope you are asking yourself or are wishing you could ask me why these plants are still wilting. Again I would say, "excellent question." I'd say maybe they don't have enough sunlight. So now we've got a lot of groups, don't we? We have fake water, fake nutrients, fake sunlight, we have fake water, fake nutrients, real sunshine, we have fake water, fake sunshine, real nutrients, etc etc. Now, at the end of our study all the plants are still wilting. What is the conclusion if we operate within the Sickness & Treatment Paradigm, define better in terms of symptoms, and ask only if our interventions can change symptoms? The conclusion is that water, sunlight, and nutrients are no good for wilting plants. Anybody who offers this care for plants would thus not be practicing evidence-based care and would be labeled a quack.

Can treating sickness ever prevent sickness or create health?

But what if we were operating within the Wellness & Prevention Paradigm? If we have evidence to show that all the plants need sunlight, nutrients and water and they got these things in sufficient amounts, did they get better if we define better as improved function and health? Yes. So why would they still be wilting? Well, perhaps because somebody has dumped diesel fuel into the soil and this toxin is getting into their systems and poisoning them.

The moral of this story is actually three-fold. The first is that we must understand that for any living creature to be well it must be sufficient in the environmental nutrients or raw materials or stimuli that it genetically requires, AND ALSO be free from toxicity, at the same time, for a period of time, before it will express its health potential. In order to express health potential an organism must have sufficiency and purity at the same time for a long enough period of time to reach homeostasis. How many humans do you think fit into this category? How many do you think get moved into this category by prescription drugs or surgery or natural "therapies" for that matter?

Clinically we can't just address one variable and expect results; this is especially true in chronic illness because all chronic illnesses are caused by a multitude of variables operating over long periods of time. There is just no point addressing only one issue. If you don't address the entire human ecosystem, and the environment in which that human ecosystem lives, then you have no chance of eliciting the expression of health or preventing illness.

Can a plant be healthy if it does not have sufficient water, sunlight, and nutrients, and is not free of toxins, at the same time for a period of time? What about humans?

I can tell you from clinical experience that a lot of times, if you're only making one change, in fact even if you're making four of five necessary changes, patients often won't see any significant clinical results until all the causal variables are addressed. This is the challenge of wellness and prevention care. In symptom care you don't have to address any causal variables, you just have to find a drug that will change a symptom or risk factor. Symptom care is quick and sexy and it fits our societal demand for quick and easy options. The only problem is that it doesn't work to produce health, it is incredibly expensive, and it causes a great deal of harm in terms of adverse effects and unaddressed causal issues that continue to drive the person toward sickness.

We live in a society now where we say, I'm going to try this and if it doesn't work in three visits or three weeks I'm going to give up or try something else. And these same people go home and eat, move, think, and interact in ways that are clearly toxic and deficient, and yet they are expecting a miracle from a practitioner. These people will give the practitioner offering a non-drug solution about three visits to fix their 25-year issue, and if it doesn't work, they go get the drug where they too often hear that anything other than drugs does not work and is not evidence-based. It becomes a self fulfilling prophesy. I will spend the rest of my life working to change this. It's my mission in life. I have seen too many lives wasted and I have done too much research to feel good about doing anything else with my life.

The second moral of our wilting plant research story is that we have to be very careful when we start talking about evidence-based care because we have to know what question was asked, we have to know what paradigm the research was conducted in. We have to know the paradigm of the researcher or the company funding the research. I can't stress how important this is and how often it is overlooked or simply not understood, especially by clinicians without a research background, which is about 99 percent of all clinicians in all healthcare fields around the world.

The third moral to this story or fable is that we have to understand that science cannot be used to tell us what questions are important to ask or which paradigm is correct. If you are so inclined you should read Thomas Kuhn's work on the importance and influence of paradigms in science, it will open your eyes very wide.[15] Reading his work clarified and solidified a great deal for me and I highly recommend it to those who have an interest in the topic. In fact I think it should be mandatory reading for every healthcare professional.

What must be understood is that science cannot give us any qualitative information. Science can only give us quantitative information. Science cannot tell us which questions to ask

"Each year the U.S. spends more than $6,700 for every man, woman, and child on what is essentially "sickness" care. In contrast, virtually every other industrial economy spends less. Greece spends less than $600 per person yet achieves superior outcomes in virtually every recognized international standard of health outcome than does the U.S. Every other industrialized economy that expends less money than the U.S. also achieves better health outcomes."

Rippe J. Lifestyle Medicine and Health Care Reform. Am J Lifestyle Med. Nov/Dec 2009

If it takes us years to develop chronic illness how long will it take to get well? Should we be expecting quick fixes from lifestyle intervention?

and science cannot determine how we should interpret and apply the results. THINK ABOUT THAT.

The two most important variables determining the value of research are the questions that are asked and how the results are interpreted and applied. Neither of these are determined by science; both are determined by the paradigm, logic, and intellect of the researcher.

Just because you have a whole bunch of science doesn't necessarily mean you asked the right questions or properly interpreted and applied the results. Only those with an infantile understanding of science actually believe that all scientists in any given field agree on which questions to ask or how to interpret and apply the results.

Can we use a scientific study or the scientific method to determine which studies are important to conduct or how to interpret and apply the results?

"The reality is that our current health care system is not truly serving our health needs. We have focused on treating illness rather than promoting prevention and wellness. The negative consequences of this sick-care system are taking a toll on our health, our economic stability and the futures of our children and grandchildren."

Richard H. Carmona M.D. M.P.H. FACS

17th Surgeon General of the United States in: Almanac of Chronic Disease, 2009 Partnership to Fight Chronic Disease

Virtually all scientific breakthroughs come from scientists asking different questions or interpreting and applying results in a different way. Breakthroughs are about paradigm not scientific methodology. To paraphrase George Bernard Shaw: "The reasonable person does what everyone else is doing. The unreasonable person does something completely different. Therefore, all progress is due to the unreasonable."[16]

Think about family history for a second. I love family history because it is just such a great way to expose the lack of logic so often applied within the gene-centric Sickness & Treatment Paradigm. It is one of the first things you learn to ask as any health care practitioner and it is just completely devoid of any recognition of the importance of environment or of epigenetics. Imagine a hunter-gatherer who is the first generation exposed to white flour, white milk and white sugar. They inevitably develop chronic illness and go see the expert in the white coat who immediately does as he or she has been trained and asks if there is any family history of whatever illness they diagnose. They answer, "No, in the history of my people there has never been obesity or diabetes" (or whatever their diagnosis is). The expert in the white coat writes down the response, offers little or no explanation as to the care of this chronic illness and of course says "take these pills."

Now as a good citizen they listen to the advice of the expert in the white coat and take their pills. Meanwhile their children consume the white milk, white flour, and white sugar and to everyone's great surprise develop chronic illness. Luckily they have the expert in the white coat. They go in and of course are asked about family history. Jackpot. This time they say, "yes my parents do have this chronic illness, how did you know?" The expert in the white coat says, "yes, I expected so, you have a genetic predisposition to chronic illness. Take these pills." You may have noticed that the actual answer to the family history question was completely irrelevant when it came to the treatment – they get pills no matter what. It's a great win-win if you get paid for prescribing, distributing, or manufacturing pills.

Think back to your last family history. Were you asked about your parents' lifestyle choices, or simply their diseases?

The problem is that family history is absurd if you are trying to equate it to genetic causes of illness because family history gives absolutely NO VALID INFORMATION regarding genetics. It does provide information about the history of patterns of illness within a family, but it does not give any information regarding the cause of these patterns of illness. Again, if you operate under the assumption that chronic illness is genetic you will will automatically assume that family history of illness equates to a history of genetic illness. No wonder they prescribe drugs and ignore lifestyle.

By the way, we also know species get genetically stronger with time not weaker so even suggesting people are developing chronic illness at ever increasing rates because of genes is contrary to both the theory of evolution and genetic science. The only relevant information or advice derived from family history is that

> "Led by a new paradigm, scientists adopt new instruments and look in new places. Even more important, during revolutions scientists see new and different things when looking with familiar instruments in places they have looked before."
>
> Kuhn, Thomas S. The Structure of Scientific Revolutions. 1962. University of Chicago Press.

which is aimed at lifestyle. *Lifestyle choices do run in families and lifestyle patterns do cause illness.*

Does family history of illness mean a history of genetic illness or a history of lifestyle illness?

But maybe we have more chronic illness because we are living longer and because we have better diagnostic ability. Not bad logic, just bad science. The data are clear. First, the largest increases in chronic illness rates are occurring among the young and the middle aged, not the elderly. Do you know that children as young as 5 and 6 are now being diagnosed with chronic illness? Did you know that they had to change the name of Adult Onset Diabetes to Type 2 Diabetes because so many children are now developing it?

Second, even if we just look at diabetes and obesity (two illnesses that are highly correlated with syndrome X or metabolic syndrome and virtually every other chronic illness, including cancer and heart disease) we see exponential increases in incidence over just the past decade. No fancy diagnostic tests are required – the technology to detect obesity (a scale and a set of eyes) or diabetes (a very simple blood test) were around for decades before the exponential increases in the incidence of these chronic illnesses.

So think about the hunter-gatherer natives that lived where you live. Imagine if we went and studied those natives before Whitey showed up. How much obesity would we have found? How much heart disease? Diabetes? Cancer? Acid reflux? ADHD? After one generation of eating like Whitey, and being socially outcast and having their self-esteem and identity destroyed, what would we have found? They would be sick. Would their genes have changed?

So when I started looking at these hunter-gatherer humans I said, "Wait a minute. Here's a bunch of humans that are living outside of captivity that are really well." Does that mean to say that they didn't get systemic infections from trauma or bug bites or snake bites? No. They got those things, but they didn't get chronic illness, even the ones that lived to a ripe old age, which was about 20 percent of them. The ones that didn't live to a ripe old age didn't die of cancer, or diabetes, or heart disease, or heart attacks, or any of those things. They died from trauma. They starved to death or died from trauma or deep infection from trauma. Hunting a mammoth with a stick can be dangerous.

Once I realized that hunter-gatherers represented a group of humans that had significantly less chronic illness, among all age groups, than industrial humans, I had to find out why. I had to discover what the difference was between healthy hunter-gatherers and sick, industrial citizens.

What is the difference between healthy hunter-gatherers and sick, industrial citizens?

You might be wondering if it is possible to study hunter-gatherers. The answer is yes, but sadly, very sadly in my opinion, that is becoming less true as the habitat and thus lifestyle of the few remaining tribes is rapidly disappearing. However there are valid data collected from hunter-gatherer tribes like the !Kung and others in Africa, the aboriginals in Australia, the natives here in North America, the Inuit up in Greenland, some of the tribes down in South America, and the tribes in Papua, New Guinea. We've actually got some great data from these people living today, although we're destroying the planet at such a rate that they're probably not going to be able to live that lifestyle much longer, their way of life is going extinct. What a tragedy, they have so much to teach us. If you have not seen the BBC series or read the book *Tribes* by Seth Godin please do so. It is an amazing insight into how we are genetically designed to live and how genetically incongruent so much of industrial life has become.

In our society, which is dominated by the Sickness & Treatment Paradigm, and by the medical, pharmaceutical and insurance industries, we have been effectively told to shut up and butt out of our own health. We have been told to leave our health to the experts. The problem is the experts are not experts in health at all, they are experts in diagnosing and treating disease and symptoms.

When it comes to your health, the truth is that you need to

become the expert because it is your day to day decisions that have the greatest impact on your health and quality of life. If you are not the expert, you have no chance. You cannot leave health to anybody but yourself, because it's your choices that are going to determine your health. You can't blame anybody else and you can't rely on anybody else.

You have to take responsibility for your health, but before you can do that you have to be given some knowledge, you have to be taught how to fish, not simply given some fish (or more likely in industrial society some highly processed, chemically-filled fish sticks). For too long now the knowledge about health has been guarded, it has been monopolized, it has been taken away from the individual and hoarded by so-called experts. This has been devastating. We have never had so little health and so much sickness. Further, we now spend trillions on medical practitioners, medical insurance, and pharmaceuticals – all this in the midst of a chronic illness pandemic.

Shouldn't expertise in the requirements for health be common knowledge? Should this not be taught to everyone rather than to a specialized few?

"While chronic degenerative diseases generally produce mortality later in life, they begin much earlier, often in childhood. This allows comparison between age-matched younger members of industrial and technologically primitive societies. Biomarkers of developing abnormality such as obesity, rising blood pressure, nonobstructive coronary atherosclerosis, and insulin resistance are common among the former, but rare in the latter."

Eaton SB, & Cordain L. Evolutionary health promotion. Prev Med 2002; 34:109-118.

Back to my question about why hunter-gatherers of all ages have more robust health and less chronic illness than industrial citizens. The more I studied the difference between hunter-gatherers (wild humans outside captivity) and industrial citizens (wild humans in captivity), the more I realized that the difference could not be attributed to genes. That was a profound realization for me and it will be a profound realization for you and it will be a profound realization for our society. My hope is that this realization will change paradigms and stimulate much more research regarding the importance of environment and lifestyle regarding human health and sickness.

Some great thinkers and scientists like Eaton and Booth and Roberts and McEwan and Schulkin and Lipton and Sterling and Goldstein and Waterland are doing just this and their research has helped me to discover the truth about why humans are so sick and what we need to do to get and stay well. Please go to the bibliography section of this book and choose to read some of the research that has brought me to my conclusions. There is just so much evidence. There are a lot of great thinkers out there who have published some amazing work that has helped me to answer the questions that I have sought answers to. I can take some credit for coming up with the right questions, but I must give all credit to the researchers who have published work that has allowed me to find the answers, or, perhaps more accurately, to discover the self-evident truths that our ancestors lived by for millenia. The more I think and study this, the more self-evident and simple it becomes.

If we want to find answers to why we are sick and how to get and stay well should we be asking gene-centric questions or lifestyle-centric questions?

Some of the most intelligent, most highly respected researchers in the world have come to the same conclusions that I have. I think what is different is that most of them are so specialized in their area that they have not put it all together into a "bigger picture", the way I have been able to do. That is changing – thank goodness. What I can say is that there is no shortage of solid, peer-reviewed scientific evidence to substantiate the conclusions I put forward in this book and there is a great deal of peer-reviewed scientific evidence to refute the current status-quo regarding healthcare research and delivery. I will share some of this research with you in later chapters. You will be in a state of disbelief about the volume of evidence that has been ignored and the lives that have been lost due to a combination of incorrect paradigm, lack of familiarity with evidence, arrogant refusal to acknowledge evidence, and greed.

There is a great deal of evidence which makes it clear that the pharmacological and surgical approach to chronic illness is not only failing in terms of health outcomes, it is so expensive that it is bankrupting individuals, corporations and governments. As you progress through the following chapters, you will read research about chronic illness rates and the human and economic cost of ignored prevention strategies and ineffective treatments that will make you at the very least shocked, but more likely outraged. Don't waste this outrage. Use it to inspire yourself to change your own health strategies and to help others do the same. Use it to improve and prolong your life and the lives of those you love.

Chapter 4
From Super Species to Sickest Species: Why Humans Have Become So Sick

And hark! how blithe the throstle sings!
He, too, is no mean preacher:
Come forth into the light of things,
Let Nature be your Teacher.

She has a world of ready wealth,
Our minds and hearts to bless
Spontaneous wisdom breathed by health,
Truth breathed by cheerfulness.

One impulse from a vernal wood
May teach you more of man,
Of moral evil and of good,
Than all the sages can.

Sweet is the lore which Nature brings;
Our meddling intellect
Mis-shapes the beauteous forms of things:
We murder to dissect.

Excerpt from The Tables Turned - William Wordsworth

Is there anything more important in your life than your health and the health of those that you love?

Health is Our Greatest Asset

I am very privileged to be able to speak all over the world and share my information about why humans have become so sick and what we can do to get and stay well. I regularly lecture to practitioners and to the general public in the United States, in Canada, in Australia and New Zealand, in Europe and soon, if I can find the time to accept the invitations, in South America and Africa. No matter where I go, there is one thing I find in common everywhere, especially in the industrial world: Humans as a species are losing their health at a great rate. The human species is getting sicker and sicker as time goes on, not healthier.

Ironically I have also discovered that everyone agrees that health is our greatest asset. Health is, quite simply, the most important thing determining the quality and quantity of our lives.

I would suggest, in fact I know, and I've spoken to tens and tens of thousands of people around the world who have agreed, that there is nothing that any of us would trade for our health, or for the health of those that we love. The tragedy is that I have never met anyone who feels that they or their loved ones are as healthy as they could be or want to be. In fact I have met thousands upon thousands who are sick and suffering and searching for answers.

The fact that we know, and openly admit, that health is the single most important thing in our lives, yet also admit that we are not expressing our genetic potential for health, happiness, and vitality, is an incongruency that we simply cannot ignore any longer. I would bet that most, if not all of you reading this, have engaged in some behaviors during the past week that you knew made you less healthy. You've also almost certainly failed to engage in some things that you knew would have made you more healthy. The same is probably true for those you love. This is what I call the great health paradox, or the apple and the donut paradox, which I will discuss in detail later.

I think that what you have just discovered, or at least became consciously aware of, is profound. Let's summarize. You have admitted that there is nothing more important than your health or the health of those that you love. You have admitted that both you and your loved ones knowingly engage in unhealthy behaviors and knowingly fail to engage in healthy behaviors. You have admitted that neither you nor your loved ones are as healthy as you'd like to be or have the potential to be.

Are you expressing your full potential for health and vitality?

You have admitted that, although health is your most important life asset, you are not expressing your full genetic potential for health, happiness, vitality, or life satisfaction. And, most significantly, you have admitted that YOUR CHOICES are significantly involved in this health paradox.

I believe that everyone's purpose is to maximize their chance to enjoy a long and happy life and to contribute to the abilities of their family and community to do the same. If we are not experiencing this and if we are engaging in activities that we know are depriving us of this experience, we have to step back and ask ourselves why. Asking why is not always easy and it is not always popular.

As I've spent the last 25 years researching and, even more so since I've spent the last 10 years traveling the world sharing that research, there has been a lot of times when it would have been more comfortable to be quiet. However, I believe with every molecule and cell in my body, as a scientist, as a clinician, and most importantly, as a father, that when you have compiled enough evidence to unequivocally support your conclusion, that it is a moral

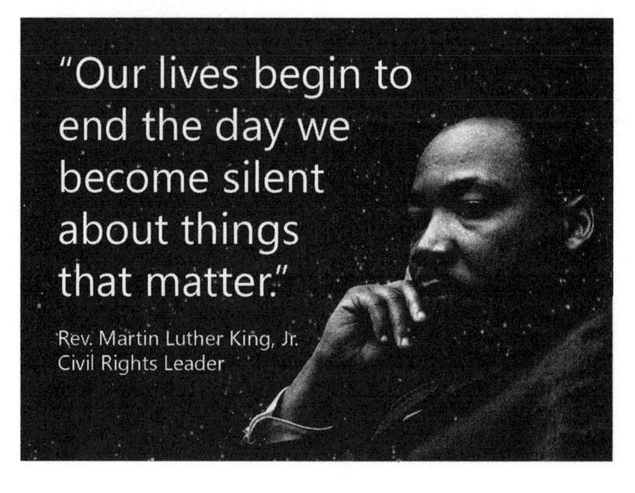

obligation to share that conclusion. This is especially true when that conclusion can save lives. I firmly believe that if you have valid information that can save the lives of those who hear and understand it that if you fail to share that information it becomes an act of immorality - by omission.

If you have information that can save lives, is it your moral obligation to disseminate that information?

As Martin Luther King said, "Our lives begin to end the day we become silent about things that matter." Health matters to me. My health matters to me and your health matters to me. This is why I refuse to be silent about what I have learned. What matters to us is what drives our behaviors. This is a very important point that will come up again and again.

My job is to get your health and your lifestyle choices to matter to you. When this happens you will change your behavior. When you change your behavior you will change your health. When you change your health you will change your life.

Just because this matters so much to me doesn't mean that disseminating this information is easy all the time. I spend a lot of time away from home, and there is nothing more important to me than being at home with my wife and children. However, at some point, we have to make a choice about what we are going to do as parents and as citizens. I believe the greatest gift we can give our children, other than loving them unconditionally and making them feel safe and loved and important, is to be good role models and to make them proud of us. We also need to leave them and their children a healthy environment, both socially and physically. If traveling the world is necessary to do that then that is what I will do and I will never regret it and neither will my children.

Herophiles said, "When health is absent, wisdom cannot reveal itself, art cannot be manifest, strength cannot be exerted, wealth is useless, and reason is powerless." He said this in 300 B.C. That is over two thousand years ago. As Mark Twain said, "Our ancestors stole all our great ideas."

> "When health is absent, wisdom cannot reveal itself, art cannot be manifest, strength cannot be exerted, wealth is useless, and reason is powerless."
>
> Herophiles

Taking Responsibility for Our Health

How many of you would agree that, in terms of your health, an apple is better than a donut, exercise is better than no exercise, and positive thoughts and relationships are better than negative ones? Unanimous, I hope. A couple of years ago I was hired to do a lecture to all of the grade five students in the local school district. It was interesting because I asked them the same questions. I asked all of these ten year olds whether an apple or donut was healthier for them. They all agreed that an apple was healthier. I then asked if exercising was healthier than not exercising. They all agreed exercising was healthier. I then asked whether happy thoughts and relationships were better than unhappy thoughts and relationships. Once again they unanimously agreed - happy thoughts and relationships were healthier. Then I asked them if they would feed their puppies soft drinks or water and they all said water. I asked them if they would feed their rabbits fresh, raw vegetables or french fries and they all said fresh, raw vegetables. Keep in mind these were ten year olds.

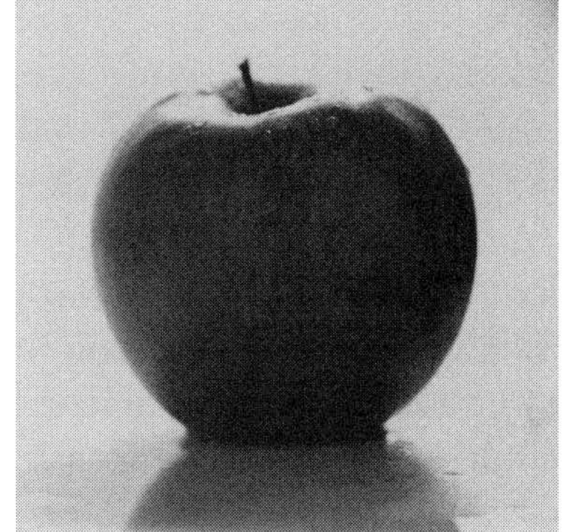

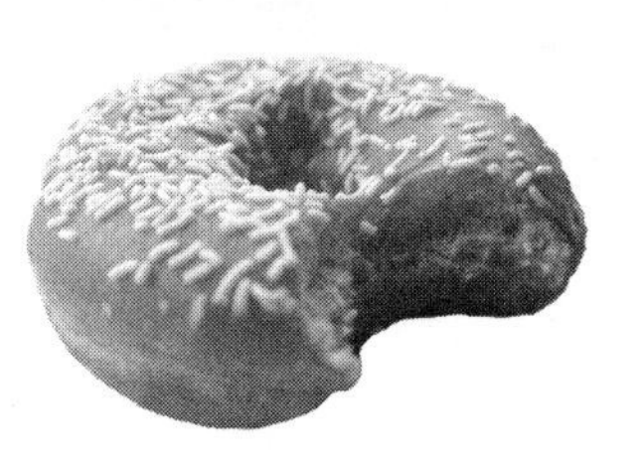

Then, I asked them what their parents and their schools fed them. Ouch.

When it comes to determining the quality and quantity of your life, is there anything more important than your health?

I asked them if they would exercise their puppies or keep them locked up inside and never give them a chance to run and play. They all agreed exercise was better.

Then, I asked them if their parents and teachers made sure they exercised every day. Ouch.

I asked them if they would give their puppies love and attention and make sure their puppies were safe and felt loved or if they would be unkind to their puppies and not be concerned with whether or not they were safe or how they felt. They all agreed that ensuring the puppies were safe and felt loved was better. Then, I asked them if they were safe and felt loved. I asked if they made sure all their schoolmates and family members felt safe and loved. I asked them how they knew if they didn't ask.

Are our children well fed, well exercised, and well loved? Whose responsibility is this?

I asked them if they could remember the last time their parents or teachers asked them if they felt safe and loved. Ouch.

The room went silent as it should have. People were really thinking, they were becoming conscious of these issues. It wasn't too complicated; the ten year olds got it. It wasn't too simple; the adults got it. It just wasn't something that they had spent enough (or any) time thinking about or acting upon - yet they all intuitively knew they should. These things are self-evident, they are part of our genetic blueprint. It is a human tragedy that we are in a culture that ignores these core issues, which are really the issues that determine the quality and quantity of our lives. My mission in life is to change this culture. This book is part of that mission.

So why don't we regularly choose the apple over the donut, exercise over no exercise, and positive thoughts and relationships over negative ones? The answer is not because on the surface we don't understand what is healthier for us, the answer is that deep down we don't really understand the devastation that poor food, lack of exercise, and unhealthy psychosocial choices cause in our lives or the devastation of missing the essential requirements from healthy food, exercise, and healthy psychosocial choices. The answer is that at a subconscious level most people really have no idea of the actual consequences of their choices.

We are marketed, literally, to death. No pun intended. We are marketed to death to believe that our choices don't really have consequences for us.

There are things that we feed our children that we would not feed our dogs. I see parents take potato chips away from their children because they're feeding it to the dog, then say, "Sweetheart, don't feed those chips to Rover, they will make him sick. These chips are for you and your friends, not for the dog." I see people taking their dogs for a walk and leaving their obese children at home to watch television. I see people arriving home, happily greeting their dogs and then being ignored by, and completely ignoring, their children.

I remember reading a news story a practitioner sent to me. The story was about a family in the United States that was feeding their dogs soda pop and potato chips and other junk food. The animal rights people actually came and took the animals away on the grounds that feeding pets this way represented an act of animal cruelty.

What is healthier, an apple or junk food? If people say they want to be healthy, why do they freely choose junk food?

The most amazing thing to me was that these people also had children. Nobody even considered that it was cruel to feed this same poison to children. Nobody acted as the advocate for the children. Horrifiying. These same kids are without doubt regularly sick and

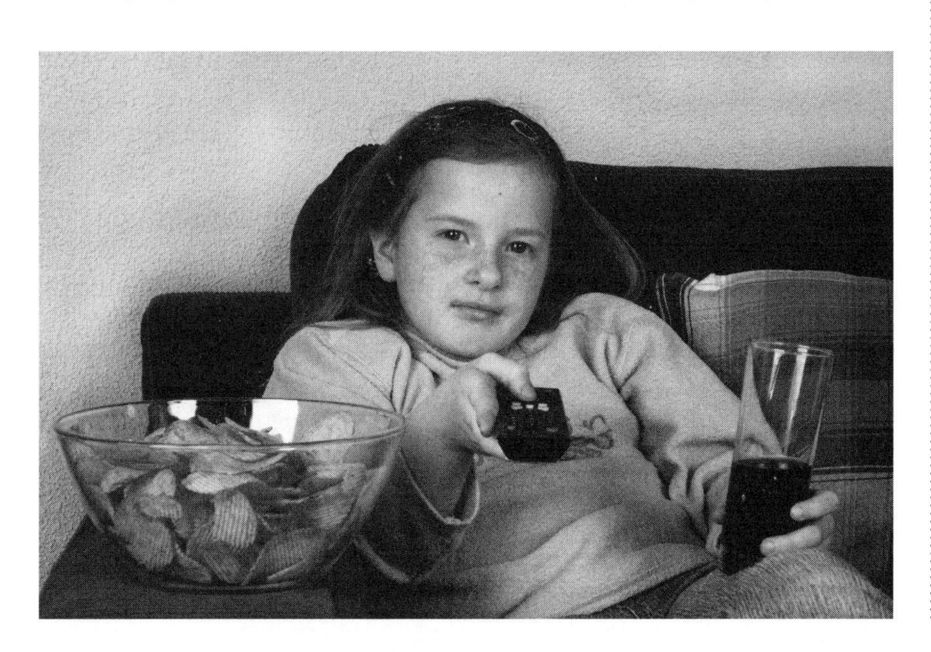

on prescriptions like antibiotics and allergy medications and in all likelihood Ritalin. *What has happened to our sense of logic?*

If the dog got sick we would ask what it ate to make it sick. If a child gets sick we ask what drug we need to prescribe. It's lunacy. The medical literature is full of data that the vast majority of antibiotic prescriptions are given for viral infections which means that the antibiotic does no good and certainly does some harm.[17] This practice also creates antibiotic resistant bacteria or superbugs. The medical literature is also full of data showing that up to 25 percent of young boys in America are prescribed Ritalin (currently 2.5 million children) and that the United States consumes over 80 percent of all Ritalin in the world.[18,19] We don't have to do it this way!

This is not evidence-based care, it is just profitable practice for people making, prescribing, and selling drugs. If it made us healthier I'd be the first to support it, it doesn't.

If it is considered inhumane to feed junk-food to pets, how is it not inhumane to feed this to children?

It makes us sicker and in the meantime the kids are still eating the junk food, sitting on the couch, playing video games, and having little to no social interaction with good role models. *How can we blame genes?* What a scapegoat and what a great belief system to instill in people if you want to sell drugs.

I speak all over the world and every time I share these anecdotes people inevitably laugh. I never laugh. I will tell you that when they begin to think about this at a conscious level, none of them find it humorous to poison a child, allow a child to become unfit, unattractive and obese, or to ignore a child. The reason they can laugh is because they don't equate the truthful consequences to their daily behavioral patterns. The truth is that they would be horrified, and you will become horrified, to discover the actual consequences of unhealthy, genetically incongruent lifestyle choices.

I find it shocking and tragic when I see what people put in their shopping carts at the supermarket. I see their overweight, hyperactive, poorly behaved children and then I see the poisons that are at the root of these issues in the shopping cart. Those poor children!

I find it inconceivable that the harmful effects of the chemicals, refined sugars, trans fats and hydrogenated fats found in so many packaged foods are well known and yet nothing is done. I find it criminal that these products are labeled and sold as food at all – they are anything but food. Food is something that is found naturally on the planet and that matches our genetic blueprint for nutritional requirements. I find it repugnant that these biochemical products made in a lab or factory are advertised, labeled, and displayed to deliberately market to children.

I find it tragic that we have unfit, overweight children and adults when exercise is free.

I find it unacceptable that daily physical activity, including walking or jogging at least a mile, some form of muscular effort, some form of balance and agility and some form of physical PLAY that is FUN, is not a mandatory part of our education and workplace environments.

Is what average people purchase at the supermarket making them healthier or sicker? What about your purchases?

I find it tragic that we have people living in educational, family, community and workplace environments where they don't feel safe, loved, and important. I find it inconceivable that our educational system does not have self-esteem training, and information about how to choose healthy thoughts and emotions as part of the core curriculum. Who cares if students can recite a fact about history or a poem or even add numbers if they don't like themselves, don't know how to be happy, and don't have healthy lifestyle habits?

I would like to take a moment now to discuss the difference between assessing blame and taking responsibility. It is important that you understand that blaming yourself for an illness or blaming someone else for theirs is both heartless and useless. Blame NEVER produces a solution and assessing blame NEVER makes anybody better. This book is NOT about assessing blame, it is about empowering individuals to take responsibility. I don't blame people for being sick, I empower as many people as possible with the available evidence about how to avoid chronic illness. I empower people with the information they need to take responsibility for their health.

Health has to be about taking responsibility and empowerment. If you don't learn to take responsibility for your health you have no chance to get and stay well.

I know I have already stated this but it warrants repeating because it is so important. You can't buy health. You also can't socialize health. You can't take health from the healthy and redistribute it to the sick. You can socialize resources for health but you can't socialize health. Health is a meritocracy, it is based on merit, you experience chronic health or chronic illness based on your effort and your choices, not based on random chance or luck or who you know. You just have no chance to express your genetic potential for health and vitality and life satisfaction unless you take responsibility for your choices. By the way, your children don't have a chance unless you teach them how to make healthy choices. Schools don't teach it, the vast majority of doctors certainly don't teach it, and governments don't teach it. You need to learn it and you need to teach it to your children and everyone else you care about – period.

Why isn't physical activity and self esteem development part of the daily school curriculum?

Just so you understand, you don't catch chronic illness, you develop it. You often earn it. You earn it with hard work, dedicated hard work. You can't get a chronic illness without years of dedicated hard work. Chronic illnesses do not arise overnight, they are not caused by one bad meal or one missed workout. Chronic illness is the product of habits not events.

Chronic illness is far too often the result of chronic suicidal lifestyle choices. You bio-accumulate the effects of your lifestyle choices and based on these choices you will either develop chronic health or chronic illness.

You just can't get chronic illness without consistently making unhealthy lifestyle choices. What is alarming is that the study of epigenetics is elucidating how our bad choices as parents can predispose our children to chronic illness because we pass on a pattern of gene expression based on the lifestyle choices we make and the environment we live in. You will learn more about this in a later chapter.

You may be getting a little uneasy at this point. Already I have challenged some of your very deep-seated beliefs about health and about healthcare. I'm not worried, I have all the evidence I need to convince you, it will just take some time for you to get through it all. I don't want you to be worried. I also don't want you to shut off the analytical part of your brain because you are feeling threatened. It is very common to feel threatened by a challenge to a deep seated belief system. Some get defensive, some get angry and some get dismissive. I've seen some get all three! If you are experiencing any of these feelings you can be sure that you are leaving the part of your brain for science and logic and entering the part of your brain for emotion. When you have evidence for your beliefs, you don't get threatened. What I mean by evidence is scientific evidence, not status quo evidence. When you are being scientific you don't get emotional, you simply ask for evidence and then you evaluate that evidence to determine whether or not you should change your opinion.

Is chronic illness something you catch or something you develop? Is chronic illness the result of an acute event or the result of chronic habits?

Real science is not about trying to prove you are right or that you know everything; science is about leaving no stone unturned in the pursuit of truth because you know for certain that you must never stop learning and questioning. Science is not about who is right; science is about giving every effort to discover what is right.

All I ask is that if you are feeling angry or defensive or dismissive then ask yourself what scientific evidence you can cite that supports your current belief system. By the way, even if you have some there is no need to get upset. Intelligent people can, and often do, disagree. They also often interpret the same data differently. There is no point arguing over reality so let's try to stick to logical interpretation of available data. The less we assume and the more we demand evidence the better. My favorite line is, "where did you read that, may I have a copy." This needs to become your mantra when it comes to health advice, regardless of the practitioner or 'expert' disseminating that advice. Regardless of who is providing it, opinion without evidence is dogma. Be aware of dogma, it is extremely prevalent.

One of the most harmful dogmatic beliefs within the Sickness & Treatment Paradigm is that lifestyle choice is not important in terms of the cause of, prevention of, or recovery from, chronic disease.

It is now controversial to suggest that people are sick because they are eating junk food or not enough fruits and vegetables. It is actually considered controversial to state that people are sick because they don't exercise enough.

Yet I will show you unequivocal evidence that our eating patterns are one of the most influential factors determining whether we get sick and whether or not we get and stay well. I will also show you evidence that exercise is not simply an optional choice to make you feel better and look better, although it will do both. Exercise is a genetically required raw material, just like oxygen, and your genes cannot produce a state of well being without daily exercise. It is no more possible for you to genetically express health without daily exercise than it is for a chimpanzee or a giraffe.

Is science about seeking evidence to prove you are right or about seeking evidence to discover what is right?

I will also show you evidence that your state of mind, whether you love and respect and forgive yourself, whether you respect and forgive others, whether or not you have a sense of self esteem, whether or not you are satisfied with your life and your relationships, whether or not you have a sense of belonging and importance within a social group or community, has a huge impact on both your emotional and physical health. I will provide evidence that without these things you cannot be well. This is not theory. I will show you the evidence.

It is an undeniable fact that our lifestyle choices and our environment are significant, in fact the most significant, determinants regarding our states of health and sickness.

It is also an undeniable fact that we as humans have been steadily changing our lifestyle choices and our environment away from what is natural and genetically congruent and healthy toward what is unnatural, genetically incongruent and unhealthy.

According to a report published by the World Health Organization, affluent populations habitually consume a diet that was unknown to the human species a mere ten generations ago.[20] Compared with the diet that fueled human evolution, the so-called affluent diet of today has much higher levels of bad fats, much lower levels of healthy fats, less than a third of the fiber intake, much lower consumption of fruits and vegetables, much higher consumption of processed foods and food additives, and much lower consumption of vitamins, minerals, and antioxidants. "World-wide, the adoption of this diet, (the whitey diet as I call it) has been accompanied by a major increase in heart disease, stroke, cancer, diabetes, and other chronic diseases."[21] Keep in mind that these are just the effects of the dietary changes. Think about the consequences of the changes to exercise and energy expenditure patterns and the increases in emotional stress levels and social isolation.

We have completely changed our environment, we have domesticated ourselves and are eating worse, moving less, and stressing out more with less social connection to help us deal with it. How can we possibly be blaming genes if, when people start to eat like us, they immediately start to get sick like us?

When it comes to determining whether we get sick or get and stay well, is there anything more important than lifestyle?

Roberts and Barnard in 2005 in the *Journal of Applied Physiology* wrote, "Currently, modern chronic diseases, including cardiovascular diseases, Type 2 diabetes, metabolic syndrome, and cancer are the leading killers of Westernized society and are increasing rapidly in developing nations."[22]

How could these illnesses be increasing rapidly in developing nations if they were caused by genes? Is it more likely that there are rampant genetic mutations occurring simultaneously in millions of individuals in developing nations or that there are rampant changes in lifestyle choices occurring simultaneously in millions of individuals in developing nations?

Billions of dollars are being spent right now trying to find the obesity gene. It just seems unbelievable to me. There is a huge market in telling you that you have no control or power when it comes to your health. And because of this, there's a huge market telling you that you have no hope and that you have to rely on somebody else to sell you something to get well.

The truth is there are no magic pills, potions or lotions. There are no quick fixes and there are no panaceas. EXCEPT LIFESTYLE. Lifestyle is the only evidence-based panacea in history. Lifestyle is the real deal, it works every time for every person. Improving your lifestyle habits makes you healthier every time, no exceptions.

Improving lifestyle habits may not completely heal every person every time, it would be misleading to suggest that lifestyle is a panacea for curing or treating chronic illness. However, improving lifestyle habits is a panacea for improving cell function and health regardless of diagnosed illness or state of health. States of cell function and health are direct effects of lifestyle habits so, by definition, improving lifestyle habits improves cell function and health.

Have the lifestyle patterns in industrial society been getting healthier or less healthy over the past 100 years?

Roberts and Barnard (2005) go on to say, "Clearly, however, there is a solution to this epidemic of metabolic disease that is inundating today's society worldwide – exercise and diet. Overwhelming evidence from a variety of sources, including epidemiological prospective cohort and intervention studies, links most chronic diseases in the world today to physical inactivity and inappropriate diet consumption."[23] That is a very powerful statement and it is published in the world's most highly respected journal for human physiology and function.

"Currently, modern and chronic diseases, including cardiovascular diseases, Type 2 diabetes, metabolic syndrome, and cancer are the leading killers of Westernized society and are increasing rapidly in developing nations."

Roberts, C.K. & Barnard, J.B. Effects of exercise and diet on chronic disease. 2005 J. Appl Physiol 98 3-30.

Boyd Eaton published a landmark article in the *American Journal of Medicine* way back in 1988. Over twenty years ago he had already gathered enough information to publish the following statements. "From a genetic standpoint, humans living today are stone age hunter gatherers, displaced through time to a world that differs from that which our genetic constitution was selected. Unlike evolutionary maladaptation, our current discord between how we live and what our genes need has little effect on reproductive success."[24] In other words, even if you eat like a suicidal maniac and move, or are sedentary, like a suicidal maniac, and think like a suicidal maniac, you're probably still going to live long enough to reproduce because chronic illnesses take time to bio-accumulate. It is most likely that you will die of chronic illness AFTER you have reproduced.

> "Clearly, however, there is a solution to this epidemic of metabolic disease that is inundating today's society worldwide – exercise and diet. Overwhelming evidence from a variety of sources, including epidemiological prospective cohort and intervention studies, links most chronic diseases in the world today to physical inactivity and inappropriate diet consumption."
>
> Roberts, C.K. & Barnard, J.B. Effects of exercise and diet on chronic disease. 2005 J. Appl Physiol 98 3-30.

Dr. Eaton goes on to say that the discordance or mismatch between what our genes require and our current lifestyle patterns act as "potent promoters of chronic illness - atherosclerosis, hypertension, cancer, diabetes, obesity, among others."[25]

How can genes, which change very slowly, be responsible for rapid increases in chronic illness rates?

Perhaps the most significant changes to our environment and to our lifestyle habits have occurred since the end of World War II and the beginning of the chemical revolution. We changed from fertilizing crops with manure to using petroleum-derived fertilizers like NPK. We began to use copious amounts of pesticides and herbicides that were developed from poison gases used in warfare. We began to chemically alter and then chemically manufacture "food". The addition of hydrogenated and trans fats became commonplace. Soon afterward artificial colors, dyes, sweeteners and flavours were developed - we came to be able to make chemical products look and taste like food. Aspartame and MSG were put into everything including baby foods. Now virtually everything we consume either contains high fructose corn syrup or some other corn or soy product. Our governments subsidize genetically modified soy crops and corn crops and we now feed

Is the human genome matched to an industrial lifestyle or to a hunter-gatherer lifestyle?

"From a genetic standpoint, humans living today are stone age hunter gatherers, displaced through time to a world that differs from that which our genetic constitution was selected.
Unlike evolutionary maladaptation, our current discord between how we live and what our genes need has little effect on reproductive success."

Eaton et al. Stone agers in the fast lane: Chronic degenerative diseases in evolutionary perspective. 1988; Am. J. Med. 84, 739-749

industrial farmed livestock corn and soy rather than grass or other foods they are genetically designed to eat. The fruits and vegetables produced by industrial farming are covered in chemicals, the soil and soil runoff are filled with chemicals, our streams, rivers and oceans are filled with chemicals, and the industrial farmed animals are so sick that they now have to be fed millions and millions of pounds of antibiotics every year.

We also started to exercise significantly less and experience a much higher level of social disconnection and emotional stress. If you look at our health status since the 1950's there is an incredible difference. I find it hard to believe that that anyone has the audacity to blame genes. The fact that health "experts" could do this is even more disturbing. Is it any wonder the current system has completely failed to prevent or solve the chronic illness pandemic or that we are in the midst of a healthcare crisis? If they would just pull their heads out of their microscopes, stop looking at genes, and start looking at the evidence regarding environment!

Way back in 1988, that is over 20 years ago, Dr. Boyd Eaton published the fact that three quarters of deaths in Industrial nations were caused by lifestyle.

This was published back in 1988 and even back then 75 percent of deaths were preventable. These deaths were caused by lifestyle, they were the result of suicide by lifestyle or, to put it more gently, they were the result of death by ignorance and misinformation. However we want to phrase it these deaths were preventable and represent a tragedy of human loss greater than any other in our history. These deaths represent millions of lost parenting and grandparenting years.

> "There is increasing evidence suggesting that the resulting mismatch between what our genes expect versus what we're delivering fosters diseases of civilization, meaning lifestyle illnesses, that together cause 75 percent of deaths in Western nations, but that are rare among persons whose lives reflect those of our ancestors.
>
> Eaton et al. Stone agers in the fast lane: Chronic degenerative diseases in evolutionary perspective. 1988; Am. J. Med. 84, 739-749

This is unacceptable; how can we continue to allow PREVENTABLE death to be the leading cause of death in our society? I can't. I refuse to accept this. Why has nothing been done to act on this information? Why has this information not been disseminated to every doctor, nurse, teacher, politician, parent and child on the planet? Paradigm and profit, that is why. Follow the dogmatic belief systems and follow the money and you will always find the answers.

What has changed since the agricultural, industrial, and chemical revolutions - our genes or our environment?

It's a fact, the vast majority of the people who are filling the hospitals, the vast majority of the people who are dying, are dying from suicide by lifestyle choice; they are dying from ignorance regarding the importance of lifestyle.

The vast majority of the money we spend on sickness care, which is deceivingly called healthcare, is being spent to treat the symptoms of chronic illness - which people are still dying from by the millions despite of all the treatments. We need people to stand up and start telling the truth. The drug ads on television are not telling the truth. People are not hearing the truth from their practitioners or from their pharmacists and they are certainly never going to hear the truth from the pharmaceutical companies.

The evidence is clear, there has been a dramatic increase in

Why has the evidence regarding lifestyle as the cause of chronic illness not been incorporated into medical education and mainstream thinking?

"There is now unequivocal evidence in the literature supporting the notion that environmental factors, including physical inactivity, defined here as less than 30 minutes of brisk walking a day, have been identified as 58-91 percent of causal factors for three of the most dominant chronic health conditions afflicting individuals in modern day America, diabetes, heart disease, and site specific cancers."

Roberts, C.K. & Barnard, J.B. Effects of exercise and diet on chronic disease. 2005 J. Appl Physiol 98 3-30.

the prevalence of chronic illnesses that were once exceedingly rare. This shift cannot be attributed to genes because the human genome is quite simply not changing at anywhere near a rate that could be responsible for this change.

A Scandinavian twin study showed that 58-100 percent of site specific cancers had an environmental origin.[26] Other important research reports that a total of 91 percent of the cases of Type 2 diabetes and 82 percent of the coronary artery cases in 84,000 female nurses could be attributed to habits of so-called high risk behavior, defined as being a little bit overweight, a diet low in fiber and Omega 3 fats, high in trans-fats and glycemic load, a sedentary lifestyle and currently smoking.[27, 28] This means that 91 percent of the cases of diabetes and 84 percent of the heart disease could have been prevented. What drug has ever or will ever be able to accomplish this? No drug, no chance, not ever.

This year alone in the United States, a million people will die of heart disease. Is that because they forgot to take their pills? No, they will take more pills than ever before in history, and they will still die.

The vast majority of deaths from chronic illness are of environmental not genetic origin. Our genes are programmed for health not sickness. It is toxic and deficient, faulty lifestyle choices, not faulty genes, that are at the root of the chronic illness crisis. Our genes do not significantly differ from our hunter-gatherer ancestors, or from modern hunter-gatherers, yet we have significantly greater prevalence of chronic illness.

The only difference between our healthy ancestors and our sick society is lifestyle choice and environment. The genes have not changed. Modern illnesses are due to environmental, not genetic factors. Modern illnesses are avoidable and modern health is attainable.

Aging is NOT Synonymous with Illness

Many people misunderstand the relationship between aging and sickness. Many think aging is synonymous with illness. Nothing could be further from the truth. There are hundreds of millions of people who are over the age of 60 and very healthy and there are hundreds of millions of people under the age of 40 who are very sick. In fact, chronic illness rates are rising most rapidly in our children and middle aged. So many of our children are obese and diabetic that they had to change the name of adult onset diabetes to type 2 diabetes.

What is the leading cause of illness, suffering, and death in industrial society?

Aging and chronic illness are are highly correlated (although this is changing as our youth become sicker and sicker) but they are not by any means synonymous. The elderly have more bioaccumulation of the effects of poor lifestyle choices and this is why we see more chronic illness as we age. Chronic illness often takes years to develop and manifest, it shows up in old age, but it has been developing for decades.

"Although our genes have hardly changed, our culture has been transformed almost beyond recognition during the past 10,000 years, especially since the industrial revolution."

Eaton et al. Stone agers in the fast lane: Chronic degenerative diseases in evolutionary perspective. 1988; Am. J. Med. 84, 739-749

The Life Expectancy Myth

One of the most commonly held misconceptions is, that because humans living in industrial society have a significantly increased average lifespan compared to those living in hunter-gatherer or primitive or developing societies, that either the industrial lifestyle, the increased drugs and surgeries that come with it, or both, should be given credit for the documented increases in lifespan. This is often provided as an argument against the superiority of the pre-agricultural or pre-industrial lifestyle and an argument for the benefits of the industrial lifestyle and industrial medicine. This is a great example of the importance of understanding the difference between correlation and cause and effect. Things that are correlated occur or change at or around the same time. Correlation does not provide any evidence of cause and effect, only of temporal relationship. A causal relationship is one where a change in one variable has been conclusively shown to reliably cause a change in another variable. The truth is that the increase in life expectancy is correlated to living in industrial society but there is absolutely not a causal relationship between increased health or increased lifespan and industrial lifestyle habits or increased access to drugs and surgeries to treat chronic illness. Let's examine this a little further so we can be sure.

Does aging cause chronic illness?

Life expectancy is now at approximately 77 years in industrial society. Although some have hailed this as a great achievement of modern medicine and modern living the reality is that it is much more an achievement of eliminating the lifestyle causes of early death from the agricultural and industrial revolutions. Obviously any change in our life expectancy cannot be due to genetics, the human genome did not significantly change during the time of documented increased average life expectancy.

Barring death from trauma or starvation, pre-industrial and pre-agricultural peoples lived long, full, active, productive lives.

When we changed from a genetically congruent, natural, hunter-gatherer way of life to a genetically incongruent, crowded, polluted, stressful, industrial way of life the human lifespan was rapidly and drastically reduced - in fact almost halved.

Average life expectancy of hunter-gatherer populations was about 42 years; life expectancy in the early towns and cities dropped to about 20 years.[29]

When methods to clean up sewage, provide ample non-rancid

foods, improve working and living conditions, and clean the polluted air and water were put into action the average lifespan quickly began to increase. This did NOT represent an increase in lifespan due to medical intervention and modern technology; it represented a decrease in early death due to environmental toxicity and deficiency. The truth is that at the time we are speaking about there was no modern medicine or technology. This rapid increase in lifespan took place before the germ theory or any drugs that could kill germs were developed. Even when you take into account later increases in lifespan the evidence is clear; the increases in life expectancy are due to two distinct factors (improved sanitation and emergency care) which have a significant effect on one very important common denominator – fewer childhood deaths. This is the variable that is actually responsible for increases in average life span.

> "Contemporary longevity reflects modern economic structure in conjunction with public health measures. It is neither an endorsement of our current individual lifestyle choices nor a valid argument against evolutionary health promotion."
>
> Eaton, Cordain & Lindeberg. Evolutionary Health Promotion: A Consideration of Common Counterarguments. Preventive Medicine 2002 (34) 119-123

If you think about how average lifespan of a population is calculated this will make perfect sense. Imagine you have a population where half the population lives to 80 years and the other half lives to only 2 years. What is the average lifespan of this population? The answer is 41 years. Even if you increased the lifespan of every elderly person in society by a few years the total effect on average lifespan would be very limited. For example, adding 5 years to the lifespan of an eighty year old only increases that lifespan by 5 years. Now, think about preventing childhood deaths. Think about preventing the deaths of a major portion of the young children in society with improved sanitation and emergency care. You would be adding decades of lifespan to each of these individuals and this would have a profound effect on the average lifespan of the entire population. This is exactly what is responsible for the increases in lifespan seen in industrial society.

Has adopting the industrial lifestyle and having greater access to drug and surgical treatments for chronic illness been responsible for the increase in average lifespan seen over the past century?

The truth is that all the drugs and surgeries administered to treat chronic illness have NOT increased lifespan. As Dr. Boyd Eaton, perhaps the world's leading expert on evolutionary health promotion, points out, despite the great deal of distributed misinformation and the subsequent widely held beliefs, "specific therapeutic medical treatments have had little impact on mortality reduction."[30]

In fact, experts predict that this generation, the most medicated and most surgeried generation of animals in the history of animals, will actually see decreases in health and lifespan.[31] The fact is that as we continue to add more drugs and surgeries, as the human genome continues to remain virtually constant, we will shorten lifespan and experience less health and less quality of life. Same genes, more drugs, more surgery, more money and less health. How is this possible? The answers will become more and more obvious as you read this book.

Did average lifespan increase or decrease as humans began to industrialize and move to crowded cities? Why?

The Pond Analogy for Aging

I often use this analogy when giving lectures. Think of two ponds in your back yard - two ecosystems. The ponds are the exact same age, you dug them on the same day. One pond you feed the genetically congruent (innate) pond diet. Some clean soil run off, some pure rain water, some organic vegetation, etc. The other pond you feed an industrial or Western pond diet. Soda, potato chips, alcohol, sugar, some pesticides and herbicides, etc.

"Life expectancy increases track more closely with economic prosperity and sanitary engineering than with strictly medical advances."

Eaton, Cordain & Lindeberg. Evolutionary Health Promotion: A Consideration of Common Counterarguments. Preventive Medicine 2002 (34) 119-123

After one year you might not notice a difference between the two ponds. After two years they may still look identical. However, after 10 years there would be a huge difference. Would you attribute this to aging? How could you, they are the same age. Would you attribute it to genetics? How could you, they shared the same species genetic profile or genome (like all humans do).

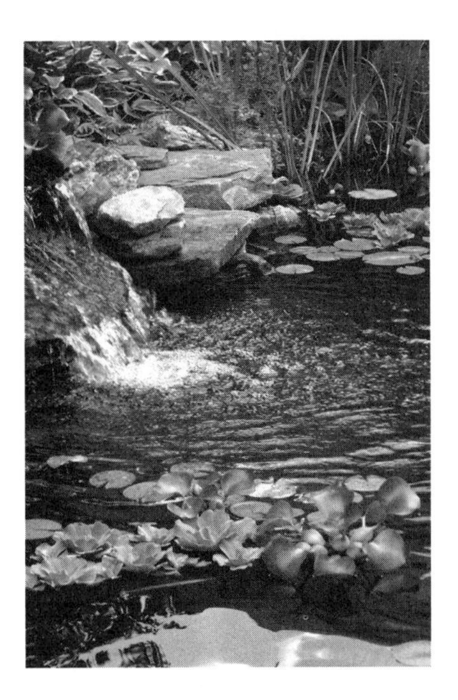

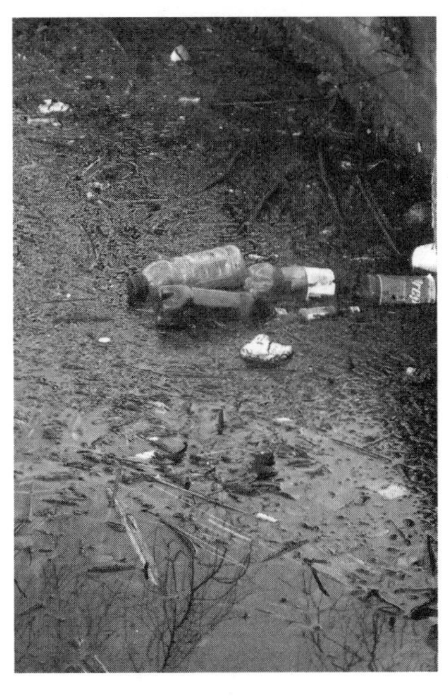

Did the significant increases in average lifespan in industrial populations occur before or after the development of the germ theory, antibiotics, and vaccines?

Now think of the difference between a healthy elderly person and an unhealthy elderly person. Think of genetically identical twins. Imagine one twin leads a sedentary life, full of emotional stress, devoid of healthy relationships, full of toxic foods, devoid of essential nutrients etc. The other twin lives a genetically congruent life, he or she eats healthy foods, exercises regularly, has high self esteem, has healthy relationships. Do you think there would be a difference in health status and/or chronic illness status by age 50 (if they both lived this long)? Could you logically or scientifically blame genes? Of course not, they have identical genes.

The aging process is not as simple as being born with a certain number of cells, and being able to keep those cells alive for 120 years. You are born and your cells turn over and divide all the time – millions and millions of cell divisions every second. So, really, what determines your rate of aging is the rate of cell division. For those unfamiliar with the reproduction process, you are formed from two germ cells, each containing half the human genome - one from your mother and one from your father. These germ cells come together when sperm infiltrates egg and they form the single celled zygote, the single celled you, and then from this cell, from this DNA, your 75,000,000,000 cells are formed, each of them genetically identical to each other. Amazing isn't it? How could we ever think our bodies are not intelligent or capable?

So what happens is that DNA from the two half cells, half the DNA from mom, half the DNA from dad, comes together to form all of your genetic code contained in that double helix in that single celled zygote. Everytime that cell divides, you have to photocopy the DNA. It's called transcription. But a photocopy is never as good as the original, is it?

It might be such a slight difference that it's barely detectable. But everytime your cells divide, you have to make a copy of that original DNA that was in your first cell, the zygote. Not only did you have to make a copy of that DNA every time you made one of your 75,000,000,000 cells, you are also making millions of copies every second as these cells continually divide. It is almost incomprehensible. So, you started with an original, then you made a copy, then a copy of the copy, then a copy of the copy of the copy etc etc. What happens is, after 120 years, the quality of the copies becomes so poor that the recipes for life cannot be read or followed and you get kidney failure or liver failure or some other failure and you die of old age. Anything in your life that speeds up the rate of cell division, that speeds up the rate at which you make copies of your DNA, also speeds up your rate of aging.

If there were two genetically identical twins and one had a healthy lifestyle and the other ate very poorly and too much, did not exercise, had low self-esteem, and had bad relationships, would there be a difference in their health status?

So genetically it appears that humans get about 120 years worth of cell divisions before our DNA, or at least some portion of it, becomes unreadable due to damage, or, in the photocopy analogy, due to lack of clarity of the recipe for life.

Let's for the sake of example say that our DNA is capable of a million accurate photocopies before it becomes unreadable. Normally, in healthy environmental conditions, it takes about 120 years to use up all these cell divisions. However, any stressors in our environment cause two things. Stressors cause an increase in the rate of cell division so that we use up our number of readable photocopies in less than 120 years. If we have a lot of stressors and double our rate of cell division we would, for the sake of this example, only live to the age of 60. The other thing stressors do is cause DNA damage so that even if we can make an accurate photocopy the recipe book or blueprint itself might have spelling mistakes or "typos" caused by this damage and thus the recipe for life is not accurate which can cause cells, tissues, organs, and systems to dysfunction.

Now in terms of stressors it is a good time to point out that one of the greatest stressors is hopelessness. If you believe you are sick because of genes you also believe that your sickness is inevitable, that your choices and efforts are meaningless. You are not only helpless but hopeless. However, if you get taught the truth, that your choices and efforts have a profound impact on your health destiny, you begin to feel empowered, you begin to feel like you can take responsibility for, and ownership of, your health destiny.

Many people believe whether they are sick or well is based on luck or random chance. Many others believe it is based on the genes they are born with. They actually believe they are born genetically programmed to express cancer, heart disease, diabetes, or some other chronic illness. What a devastating thing to believe!

Believing this means you have no power, it means you have no control, it means your life is predetermined and that your efforts are irrelevant. There is no greater lie and no greater stressor.

Why do we age if we constantly produce new cells throughout our lifespan?

When people learn just how much control they do have, when they learn just how much power they have to determine their own destiny, they start to live their lives with less of a burden and with much greater hope and self-esteem. Genes do not determine our health, genes determine our species type. Our choices determine our health and we have the power to make healthy or unhealthy choices. We have free will but it is very unlikely we will exercise that free will if we believe that our choices are irrelevant because our lives are genetically predetermined at birth. When people who believe that genes control their health get sick, they've taken on the role of victim, they don't invest any energy into taking control of their own health. Why would anyone invest energy in lifestyle change if they believe their states of health and sickness are genetically predetermined?

Once again we are brought back to the importance of paradigm and asking the right questions. We have to find the right answers to the right questions. We must find the truth regarding why humans have become so sick with chronic illness and then, and only then, can we discover what humans need to do to get and stay well. We will never know what is required to get and stay well until we know what is causing us to get sick. Incorrect, dogmatic assumptions regarding why we get sick, assumptions that we are sick due to genes, are preventing us from finding solutions to get and stay well.

Right now, without question, the prevailing belief system and the medical/pharmaceutical old science view is that we are sick with chronic illness because of bad genes, bad cells, or bad luck. Sometimes, you can throw bad germs in there, but really, with chronic illness, it is almost always assumed that bad genes and/or bad cells are to blame.

The idea that the chronic illnesses that are killing 80 percent of our population are genetically predetermined is the prevailing belief system and this belief system drives medical education, research, and clinical care.

What effect does chronic exposure to environmental or lifestyle stressors have on lifespan?

If this belief is true, which people obviously believe it is, then that means there is no possibility of wellness or prevention because if illness is genetically predetermined, there can be no hope of any cure or any prevention. It's genetically predetermined. It's inevitable. It's a hopeless belief system that has spawned a hopeless healthcare system. Our health care system based on diagnosing and treating illness and symptoms only makes sense if chronic illness is genetically predetermined. If this were true, it would make perfect sense to spend all our time, money, resources, and intellect looking for ways to diagnose and treat the inevitable illnesses that are coming our way. It wouldn't make any sense to spend any money or energy on wellness and prevention because these are a waste of time and resources if illness is genetically predetermined.

Clearly this is why medicine spends less than three percent of its resources on wellness and prevention and the truth is that this three percent is comprised almost entirely of what is called early detection (mammograms, pap smears, colonoscopies etc). These tests don't prevent anything![32]

Understanding Genetics, Lifestyle, and Health

I recently sat down and interviewed Dr. Bruce Lipton Ph.D., author of the books *The Biology of Belief* and *Spontaneous Evolution* (you can order copies of his books at www.brucelipton.com or you can order an audio copy of this interview at www.wellnessandprevention.com). I found it an incredible experience on several levels. First, when I contacted Dr. Lipton I of course offered to pay for his time. He insisted that, as he was coming to my area to give a lecture at a hospital anyway, he would not require any compensation. Keep in mind this is one of the busiest lecturers in the world! I had a series of questions ready to ask him, I was filming the interview for a documentary I am working on and I wanted to make sure I got everything covered that I felt was important. To my amazement as soon as the camera man said 'action' we just began to talk as old friends or perhaps more accurately like two excited explorers discussing their recent discoveries.

What was really amazing to me is that we had started from two opposite ends of the biological spectrum and both come to the exact same conclusion – it's not genes, it's the environment.

If people believe that whether they get sick or stay well is genetically predetermined, why would they invest any time, energy, or resources into lifestyle for wellness and prevention?

Dr. Lipton began as a cellular biologist studying DNA in stem cells and I began my search from the viewpoint of biological ecosystems or species and the environment. I started from the level of species living in ecosystems or environments and worked my way down to DNA and he started from DNA and worked his way up to species and their ecosystem environments. What we discovered was that we had been reading a lot of the same research and coming to a lot of the same conclusions. To use a great quote from one of Dr. Lipton's instructors that he included in his book *The Biology of Belief* - "It's the environment stupid". This is the inevitable conclusion we have both come to and we are certainly not alone – the entire field of epigenetics is based on this same view.

Decades ago Dr. Lipton was studying stem cells. He would put genetically identical cells into petri dishes and then he would change their environments (the lifestyle choices of the cells) and what he found was that cells got sick in sick environments and cells got healthy in healthy environments – EVEN THOUGH THEIR GENES REMAINED CONSTANT. He also found that when he took these genetically identical cells and put them with different tissues they morphed, via changes in genetic expression, into that tissue. In other words, as an example, if he put undifferentiated stem cells with heart tissue the stems cells turned into heart cells. If he put undifferentiated stem cells with pancreatic tissue the stem cells turned into pancreatic cells. Now it does not take a Ph.D. in biochemistry or physiology to figure out that heart cells look and function VERY differently from pancreatic cells. The take home point here is that the stem cells were genetically identical to each other and so were the heart and pancreatic cells.

The thing that determined their structure and function and whether they were sick or well was THE ENVIRONMENT THEY LIVED IN and not their genetic code.

Stem cell research is not research about the importance of genes, it is research about the importance of the environmental determination of gene expression. It is research regarding how the EXPRESSION of genes is determined by the environment and how health and function are determined by the expression of genes – in other words our health is determined by the environment. This is really a description of epigenetics which we will discuss in more detail later.

Is early detection a valid strategy of prevention? Is it possible to prevent something that has already been detected?

I have always taught that genes are recipe books. Genes contain the recipes for life, they contain the codes or recipes for our cells to create proteins and protein products like enzymes and hormones and tissues.

Genes contain the recipes that allow us to use proteins to create the structure, biochemistry, and physiology that is best suited to survive and thrive and reproduce in any given environment. However, the main point to understand is that genes do not control themselves.

Genes are passive storage units of information. Genes are not turned on or off, they are inanimate. Genes are simply available to read or not available to read.

In other words the page with the recipe for any particular biochemical or physiological or structural "dish" is either available to read or not. What determines this availability is NOT the genome, it is the epigenome, the coating that covers the DNA and determines which recipes are available to be copied (transcription) and taken to the kitchen to create a dish (translation) - a hormone or enzyme etc that controls structure and function in the body and brain. So think of your genes as a recipe book. Your genes are passive. They just sit there. What is required is a shopper that chooses fine ingredients based on the ingredients list found in that recipe book for the dish we call health.

The genes are NOT the shopper, the genes have no control over what ingredients are supplied; the genes simply determine which ingredients are required to successfully create the dish called survival and health. The cells of your body act as the master chefs, the recipe is translated in the cytoplasm of your cells at the kitchen called the ribosome. The recipe and the skills of the chefs virtually never change; the recipe has been developed and perfected over millions of years and the chefs together with their ancestors have had millions of years of experience cooking the same dishes. The ingredients are your lifestyle choices and it is up to you, the shopper, whether you supply ingredients that match the genetic recipe book instructions (healthy choices, genetically congruent choices) or whether you choose ingredients that do not match the genetic recipe book instructions (unhealthy choices, genetically incongruent choices).

Is stem cell research providing evidence for the importance of gene code or environment?

For thousands of years humans had few choices other than those which were matched to the ingredients set out in the recipe book. However, since industrialization, and especially since the end of WW II, humans have not only had an ever increasing number of lifestyle choices available that were not matched to the ingredients set out in the recipe book, we have actually developed a society that makes such incongruent, unhealthy ingredients choices more convenient than the healthy ones. We have developed a culture whose economy is almost entirely based on the marketing and sale of these unhealthy choices and a sickness care system that markets and sells the diagnosis and treatment of the effects of these choices.

We live in a society that teaches you to blame the recipe book and the chef instead of the person responsible for supplying the ingredients. We live in a society that has a sickness care system that diagnoses the problem after the dish comes out of the oven because they believe the quality of the dish is based solely on the recipe book and the chef and not the ingredients. Even more illogically, they have no proof that the recipe or the chef is faulty, they just assume this because they believe that the recipe and chef determine the outcome of the dish and thus believe, by deduction, that if the dish is faulty the recipe and/or chef must also be faulty.

Not a bad hypothesis but it is WRONG. Sadly, our entire healthcare system is based on this faulty premise, on this Central Dogma that states that the gene or the recipe book or chef are the sole determinants of health and sickness.

Do genes control themselves? Are genes the recipe book or the chef?

Dr. Lipton has taught the exact same concept but he uses the analogy of a blueprint instead of a recipe book. To quote Dr. Lipton from the interview we did together, "Here's what a gene is, it's a blueprint. It's a molecular blueprint that is used to make the protein building blocks of the body and the proteins give us our structure and our behavior so our characters are associated with the proteins and the DNA is a blueprint to make proteins. BUT, If you go to an architect's office and they're working on a blueprint and you lean over that architect's shoulder and say, "Excuse me. Is that blueprint on or off?" That architect is going to look at you and they are going to say, "what are you talking about? A blueprint is not on or off." Well, this is what the new science has finally come around to understand after 50 or more years of just tacitly agreeing that genes turn on and off. They've finally come to the truth; genes do not turn on and off. Genes are passive blueprints." Of course in Dr. Lipton's analogy you would be the person responsible for the supply of the construction materials. Isn't it amazing that we were both traveling the world teaching the exact same concepts using these two analogies? Now you know why I was so giddy during the interview. I felt good to have my conclusions validated by such a renowned expert and, as importantly, such a gentleman. Thank you Dr. Lipton.

Dr. Lipton and I both like to point out that we are certainly not alone in our conclusions. Recently there has been a lot of research published on the importance of gene expression vs gene code. In fact there is an entire scientific field – epigenetics – devoted to studying gene expression. I think the landmark study in this area was performed by Jirtle and Waterland in 2003.[33] Here is a brief description of their landmark experiment and some of their findings.

Jirtle and Waterland conducted an experiment on Agouti mice. Agouti mice are considered prize research mice because they have a gene which apparently causes them to get overweight, and to get cancer, and diabetes, and die early. Let me say that again. The reason these mice are so prized is because all these scientists who conduct research within the gene centric Sickness & Treatment Paradigm conclude that, because these mice get sick due to genes just like humans do, they are great subjects to use to figure out new drugs to treat human genetic diseases like cancer, obesity and diabetes.

As the article summarizing their experiment points out, "When Agouti mice breed, most of the offspring are identical to the parents, yellow, fat as pincushions, and susceptible to life-shortening disease."[34] You should also be aware that these mice have reliably produced sick, disease ridden offspring in research labs for thousands of mice generations. These mice have consistently suffered from cancer, obesity and diabetes, and experienced early death for generation upon generation and the most highly funded scientists and cancer researchers in the world have not been able to cure these mice or stem the pandemic of chronic disease in these mice. Keep in mind what paradigm these researchers were operating within and ask yourself what they believed to be the answers to why the mice were sick and how to get them well (or treat their sickness).

Who is responsible for supplying the ingredients set out in the genetic recipe book?

The article goes on and reports that, "The parent mice in Jirtle and Waterland's experiment, however, produced a majority of offspring that looked altogether different. These young mice were slender and mousy brown. Moreover they did not display their parents' susceptibility to cancer and diabetes, and they lived to a spry old age. The effects of the Agouti gene had been virtually erased."[35] They accomplished this with one experiment conducted over a few weeks. What did they do? Something so radical, you will not believe it. They changed the diet of the pregnant mice.

Why had all the billions of dollars of research funds and all the incredible scientific minds that had been studying these mice not been able to produce this result in all the years of research? Paradigm. They had just assumed that genes were the cause and because of this they had completely ignored the environment.

The most highly respected and most highly funded researchers around the world had not even considered the environment of the mice.

Would it be logical to ask an architect if a blueprint was turned on or off? Would it be logical to ask a chef if a recipe was turned on or off? Would it be logical to ask if a gene was turned on or off?

"The parent mice in Jirtle and Waterland's experiment, however, produced a majority of offspring that looked altogether different. These young mice were slender and mousy brown. Moreover they did not display their parents' susceptibility to cancer and diabetes, and they lived to a spry old age. The effects of the Agouti gene had been virtually erased."

Watters, Ethan. DNA is not Destiny: The New Science of Epigenetics Rewrites the Rules of Disease, Heredity, and Identity. Discover Nov 2006

They studied generation after generation of mice that kept producing fat, yellow, diabetic, cancerous offspring that died young. It took some researchers with a different paradigm, who were most certainly looked at as crazy quacks, to come along and say, "Why don't we change the diet of the pregnant mice to a more genetically congruent diet for mice and see what happens?" They didn't even get them exercising, they just changed the diet, and look at the result! Paradigm is everything because paradigm determines what questions we will ask and in research the question is everything. If your paradigm is that genes determine illness, and the solution is to find treatments for these genetically predetermined illnesses, you will never do an experiment on lifestyle. BUT, if your paradigm was that gene expression, as determined by the environment, determines health and illness, then you would focus completely on the environment and lifestyle. Same mice, same genes, MUCH different result.

The article goes on to point out that, "All of these discoveries are shaking the modern biological and social certainties about genetics and identity. Genes as fate had become conventional wisdom. Through the study of epigenetics, however, that notion at last may prove outdated.

Sickness & Treatment Paradigm

Genetically Determined Health and Sickness

GENOME

BIOCHEMISTRY & PHYSIOLOGY

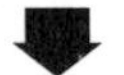

HEALTH OR SICKNESS

QUALITY & QUANTITY OF LIFE

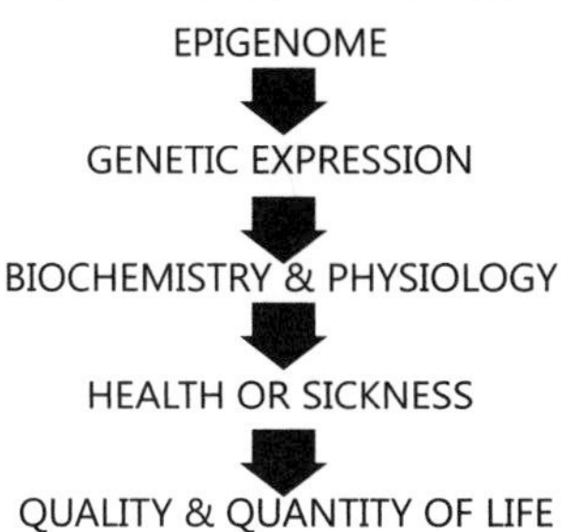

Suddenly, for better or worse, we appear to have a measure of control over our genetic legacy. Before, it was believed that genes predetermined outcomes. Now, everything we do – everything we eat or smoke can affect our gene expression and that of future generations. Epigenetics introduces the concept of free will into the idea of genetics."[36]

Are the billions of dollars being spent on cancer research funding studies looking for genetic causes and drug treatments or environmental causes and lifestyle interventions and prevention?

The authors clearly point out that genes, although they are the recipe or instruction book, are not the chef or the contractor. "Our DNA, specifically the 25,000 genes identified in the Human Genome Project is now widely regarded as the instruction book for the human body. But genes themselves need instructions for what to do, and where and when to do it. These instructions are found not in the letters of the DNA itself, but on it in an array of chemical markers and switches known collectively as the epigenome that lie along the length of the double helix." [37]

The epigenome is the proteins that lie on top of the DNA, and these proteins determine which genes are available to be copied or translated. The epigenome protein coating determines which recipes can be copied and taken to the kitchen. The thing that determines which genes or recipes are covered or uncovered is NOT the genes, it is signals from the environment. The genes themselves don't change; the genes stay the same from birth to death in any individual. But your health status can go from a 10 to an eight, to a seven, to a six, and actually come back up. The genes are the constant, the recipe is a constant, it is the ingredients that change the quality of what is produced.

It gets worse. You can mess up your grandkids. We are now learning that we bioaccumulate and pass on the negative effects of toxic and deficient lifestyles and environments in our epigenome. Our kids are being born with epigenetic patterns that reflect those of their parents.

We are now producing the sickest generation of children in the history of the human species. We have more kids with obesity and diabetes and cancers and acne and ADHD and depression and anxiety than ever before in history.

We are producing the sickest generation of children our species has ever seen. This is because we can pass on epigenetic patterns to our offspring. This makes perfect sense if you think about it. If a child is in the womb during a time of drought or low food consumption or severe heat or cold then it would make sense for any advantageous gene expression adaptations to be passed on to the offspring. The problem now is that we are not passing along advantageous adaptations, we are passing along adaptations to sedentary living, to high sugar diets, to emotional stress. These epigenetic changes are making our offspring more susceptible to the chronic disease we have developed. This makes perfect sense too. If chronic illness is a gene expression issue, an epigenetic issue, and if we can pass along epigenetic changes to our offspring, then sick adults should produce sick offspring. This is EXACTLY what is happening.

"The even greater surprise is the recent discovery that epigenetic signals from the environment can be passed on from one generation to the next, sometimes even several generations. What's eye-opening is a growing body of evidence suggesting that the epigenetic changes wrought by one's diet, behavior, or surroundings can work their way into the germ line and echo far into the future. Put simply, as bizarre as it may sound, what you eat or smoke today could affect the health and behavior of your great grandchildren."

Watters, Ethan. DNA is not Destiny: The New Science of Epigenetics Rewrites the Rules of Disease, Heredity, and Identity. Discover Magazine. November, 2006

What is the prevailing paradigm amongst most cancer researchers? What do they believe is the cause of cancer?

However, if you

believed illness was caused by genes, and you knew that the environment cannot change genes (remember that your genome or gene code does not change, only the expression of your genes changes according to your environment), then you would always assume the sick parents passed on a sick gene which caused the sick children. This has become a self-fulfilling prophesy!

There are three studies, two published in the *New England Journal of Medicine* and one published in the journal Cell, which I have found very useful in helping change deep seated false beliefs regarding the cause of cancer, and other chronic illnesses for that matter. Should this information change your beliefs or your paradigm ask yourself if who you have considered to be "experts" have been correct or incorrect. Ask if it is not possible, in fact highly probable, in fact certain, that if these experts have been incorrect about why we are sick, that they have also been incorrect about what we need to do to get and stay well. These are fundamentally important questions, especially if you have a blind faith or belief in the current system. Now, let me share these three paradigm changing studies with you.

Why are our children getting sick with chronic illness at younger ages than we did?

In Denmark they keep a very detailed register of genetic origin for their citizens. Researchers there conducted a study looking at more than a thousand adopted children. In other words they conducted a study on children who had no inherited genes from the parents who raised them; there was no biological or genetic connection between the parents and the children.

What they found was that when one of these adoptive parents died of cancer before the age of fifty the rate of cancer death among the adoptive children of these parents increased by 500 percent. [38]

No genetic connection, just lifestyle connection. Now, what are we told about family history? We are told that if our parents have an illness we are more likely to get it because we have probably inherited the genes that caused it. I have been screaming about this for years.

The truth is that family history tells us that illnesses run in families, it does NOT provide any information about why this is occurring. Most assume it is an issue of genetics but it is NOT. It is an issue of lifestyle. We learn how to eat, move, think, and socially interact from our parents. We have many of the same chronic environmental

"We show here that EE (enriched environment) leads to a remarkable suppression of cancer proliferation in all three models tested, even when delayed until the tumor was well established."

Cao L, et.al. Environmental and Genetic Activation of a Brain-Adipocyte BDNF/ Leptin Axis Causes Cancer Remission and Inhibition. Cell. 2010 Jul 9;142(1):52-64.

and lifestyle stressors.

Let's now look at the second paradigm changing study. A study conducted at the Karolinska Institute in Sweden (where Nobel Prize candidates are selected), looked at cancer rates among genetically identical twins.[39] In other words they looked at people who had IDENTICAL genes. Guess what they found? They found that having the EXACT SAME genes was not the predictive variable determining cancer. The authors conclude, "Inherited genetic factors make a minor contribution to susceptibility to most types of neoplasms (cancers)." By far the greatest determinant of who develops or does not develop cancer was the environment or lifestyle.

If chronic illness is not genetic can we pass it on to our children?

The third paradigm changing study is perhaps the most exciting and important research demonstrating that our daily living environments significantly affect both our chances of developing chronic illness and our ability to heal ourselves from it. These researchers, Cao et al. conducted a landmark study that showed that when mice were put into a more natural or genetically congruent environment they showed significantly less tumor growth and significantly increased remission compared to mice in a less natural, less genetically congruent environment.[40] Interestingly the findings showed that increasing opportunity for normal exercise and socialization increased learning and memory, immune function, improved body composition, improved insulin metabolism, improved leptin levels, and resulted in an overall increase in health.

The healthy environment got genetically expressed as healthier physiology. Having healthier or normal physiology allowed the innate healing abilities of the mice to shrink the cancer tumors. You could not get a greater endorsement for the Wellness & Prevention Paradigm or for the importance of lifestyle as the foundation of healthcare.

These findings have great implication for cancer research. If we know that a genetically congruent environment can actually result in the healing of established cancers we must acknowledge this and apply it to the interpretation and application of current research. How much of the survival from cancer is due to the support of family and friends as opposed to the treatments? When one considers how much more love and attention a cancer patient receives, how much more conscious they become of lifestyle choice, how they often are removed from stressful jobs, and how many other lifestyle and environmental improvements occur in their lives, one must also consider what part this plays in recovery. This, combined with all the other available research regarding the importance of environment and lifestyle, at the very least demands further investigation. If they don't control for any of these factors in cancer treatment research how can they ever know what percentage of the results are due to these factors? Love and support and lifestyle changes are free and they are also free from devastating side effects. How can this not be the topic of rigorous investigation? Paradigm and profit?

If medicine has been wrong about the cause of the chronic illness pandemic is it logical to believe they have been correct about the solution?

I was recently speaking at a convention addressing a room full of practitioners. As I was speaking about this topic one of the practitioners raised his hand and asked the following question. Actually he didn't ask the question he made a statement of what he thought was fact which he thought refuted my conclusions. He stated that medical interventions are able to keep genetically weak humans alive so in effect we are weakening the gene pool and thus genes can be responsible for chronic illness. He stated that the natural laws of evolution no longer apply and thus my argument was not sound.

The nice thing about not trying to be right but simply trying to find out what is right is that you ask yourself as many questions as possible. I am always asking myself questions and always trying to find information that might change my views.

The truth is I had asked myself this question years earlier. Rather than answering the question I decided, like I almost always do, to simply ask this person the same series of questions I had asked myself. I knew that if I asked him the same questions he would get the same answers.

> "Nature's biological imperative is simple: No intelligence or ability will unfold until, or unless, it is given the appropriate model environment."
>
> Eric Jensen 'Brain-Based Learning. The Brain Store 1995 San Diego, CA USA

The first thing I asked him is if he accepted the fact that over the last 100 or even over the last 50 years that chronic illness rates were rising exponentially on a per capita or per person basis. Since I had just shared the data and since this is really common knowledge for anyone in healthcare the answer was of course - yes.

Do genetically identical twins develop the same cancers or other chronic illnesses if they don't share the same environment? Do adopted children develop the same cancers or other chronic illnesses as their adoptive parents?

I then asked him if he thought it was possible that millions of people had a simultaneous genetic mutation or genetic change. He said of course not. I then asked him if he understood what would be required to spread "weak genes" through a population. I asked him, for example, that if he thought a "weak gene" was responsible for the exponential increases in cancer or heart disease or obesity or diabetes over the past 50 or 100 years how this gene got disseminated through the population. He just look puzzled - he started thinking.

I then asked him to imagine that I was the most promiscuous man alive. I then asked him how many offspring I could have passed my "weak gene" to in 50 years or even 100 years. I then asked him how many more individuals are getting chronic illness now than 50 or 100 years ago. He just looked at me and tapped the palm of his hand on his forehead and said "I just never thought of it that way." What he meant of course was that he had never asked those questions.

I thanked him for his question (even though it started as a statement of 'fact') and said that this was my goal. My goal was to get practitioners to ask the right questions so they could come up with better solutions for their patients.

My goal with this book is to get you to ask better questions so that you can come up with better solutions for you and your loved ones. The question is EVERYTHING. What determines the questions we ask is our paradigm.

If you have a gene-centric Sickness & Treatment Paradigm you will ask sickness and treatment questions. If you have a lifestyle-centric

Wellness & Prevention Paradigm you will ask wellness and prevention questions. The goal of this book is to teach you how to think, ask, and act within the Wellness & Prevention Paradigm.

What I really want YOU to begin to understand is that whatever state of health you are in right now is, in fact, the genetic expression of your environment. Your health is the genetic expression of your thoughts and social interactions, it's the genetic expression of your food choices, it's the genetic expression of your exercise and energy expenditure patterns. It is the genetic expression of how you eat, move, and think and the environment you live in. As I have been teaching for over a decade, our chronic state of health is the genetic expression of our chronic lifestyle choices.

Chapter 5
The Genetic Expression of Illness: Understanding Stressors, Adaptive Physiology, and Sickness

"Note that "adaptation" refers simply to the resetting of response sensitivity to a signal (stressor). Although it may turn out badly over time, the outcome is not caused by any low level error or defect."

"The allostasis model clearly identifies a paradox: people are dying, but their internal regulatory mechanisms are intact. So where should we intervene?"

Peter Stirling Ph.D. – Department of Neuroscience, University of Pennsylvania

Why We Get Sick - Toxicity And Deficiency

Let's now begin to look more deeply into the cause of illness, let's begin to develop an understanding of the physiology of sickness. What we have to figure out now is why our genes would genetically express illness instead of health. As you will soon learn it is all about stressors. Stressors, or genetically incongruent ingredients or environments do what? Stressors increase the rate of cell division and increase the rate of aging and increase the rate of cell damage. Any time you eat, move, think, or interact in ways that are toxic and deficient, that are genetically incongruent, you increase your rate of cell division and cell damage and you also increase the struggle of day to day life. You have a worse, shorter life when you do not choose a healthy lifestyle.

I want to remind you that it is unscientific to blame lifestyle illnesses on aging. There's only one thing that aging causes, and that's getting older. There is some degeneration with aging, of course, but most of the sicknesses that many assumed were due to aging are not due to aging at all, they are due to the bioaccumulation of the effects of stressors, of genetically incongruent lifestyle choices and environments. Remember the pond analogy for aging.

Think of all the animal species becoming endangered or going extinct. Think of the orca whales in Puget Sound and in the Juan de Fuca Strait where I live. Now, we know that, as they get older, these beautiful marine mammals bio-accumulate more and more toxins such as PCBs and fire retardants (shockingly PCB use has been banned for decades but the PCBs do not breakdown and have infiltrated the entire ecosystem). So when the orcas become sicker as they age, should we conclude that it is because of old age, or because they have bio-accumulated poisonous toxins? Well certainly the answer is obvious to any marine biologist and to any logical layperson.

I strongly dislike and disagree with the concept of anti-aging, I find it both insulting and unnatural. A better concept would be anti-premature aging. Normal aging is a wonderful, beautiful part of life, and it's only in this ridiculous culture that we don't honor our elderly.

In part this is likely because our elderly are often very sick and can indeed become a burden. But our elderly are sick because of the way they lived in the years prior to becoming elderly, not simply because they are old. If you look at native cultures, hunter-gatherer cultures, genetically congruent cultures, the elderly weren't overweight, lying around with tubes hanging out of them. They weren't a burden to have around the teepee or the longhouse or the hut; they were a valuable asset. Do you know what their greatest asset was?

Can knowledge and skills regarding how to live a healthy lifestyle ever become outdated or unimportant to pass on from elders to younger generations?

Their greatest asset was that they helped raise the children and they passed on the most significant information that we can pass on from generation to generation - how to eat, move and think and how to be a valuable, contributing member of a tribe.

We can make all the excuses we want, we can say that society is changing so fast now. We have computers and cars and television and cell phones. The truth is that when my grandmother was born she rode in a horse and buggy as a child and by the time she was a grandmother humans had landed on the moon. We can use this excuse to claim that her knowledge and skills became irrelevant in a fast changing world. That's garbage. You know what's relevant? How to eat, move and think, and how to love one another, and how to have a family raise a child. That is timeless wisdom and it is applicable to every generation. It is this generation's skill set and wisdom for living that is lacking. Technology is not genetically congruent. It can't build a healthy human or a healthy family or a healthy society. Technology can certainly provide advantages but we can, and have, thrived as a species without it. We have more technology than ever before yet we are getting sicker and sicker.

What we cannot thrive as a species without is knowledge about how to live a healthy lifestyle and how to build healthy children and families and societies.

For the last few generations in industrial society we have been told health should be left to experts rather than to individuals. We have been convinced that experts in sickness and disease will miraculously be able to keep us healthy. This is like depending on experts in bankruptcy to provide information about how to build wealth; it is illogical and dangerous. As a society we have now reached the dangerous point where we are unable to pass on the wisdom of how to eat, move and think to our children. Think of breast-feeding, or basic first aid, or basic outdoor survival skills.

Can technology build a healthy human being or a healthy family?

Most people pay more attention to which car they will buy than the resources they provide for the health of themselves and their families. It's time to change this.

It is time to figure out why we have made such bad choices and how we can start to make some good choices. Our lives and the lives of our loved ones depend on this.

Toxicity and Deficiency – The Root Causes of all Illness

There are two categories of stressors that cause cells to move away from a state of healthy function and toward a state of sick cell function (away from 10 on the scale of cell function and health). These two categories apply to all living organisms. These two categories of stressors are the explanation regarding why we have become so sick with chronic illness. The first category is toxicity; something toxic has entered into your ecosystem, into your cells. Toxins are defined as those things which force a state of adaptation. Toxins can be physical trauma, poisons, chemicals, pollutants, drugs, bacteria, viruses or even toxic thoughts and relationships.

The second category is deficiency; you are not supplying your ecosystem something that is genetically required for healthy cell function. You are deficient in something that your cells genetically require to function properly. You are not putting an essential nutrient or raw material into your ecosystem which is a genetic requirement for you to express your health potential - to move toward 10 out of 10 on the scale of cell function or homeostasis. Toxicity and deficiency are the root causes of all chronic illness in all living things. Stop and think for a moment. Try to think of any illness that is not caused by either or both of these two variables.

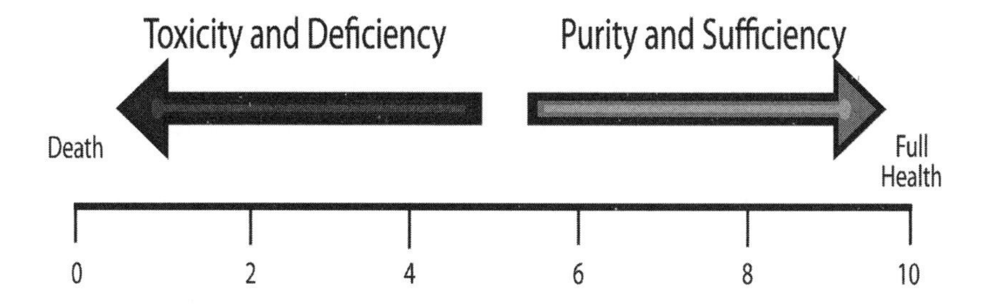

Why would your cells move away from health and enter a state of adaptation?

You might be thinking that Down's Syndrome or Cystic Fibrosis or other genetic illnesses are exceptions to this. You may or may not be correct. I would hypothesize that there was a toxicity and/or a deficiency that caused the genetic change in the first place or that there was a toxicity or deficiency that was responsible for a breakdown in the innate mechanisms in place to detect and correct unhealthy genetic change. Either way, the most important fact to be aware of is that less than three percent of all sickness can be attributed to a hereditary genetic cause.[41] A genetic illness is an illness that is defined by the absence or presence of a particular gene or genes. If you have the genes that define that genetic illness you have the illness 100 percent of the time.

Anytime someone is trying to call an illness a genetic illness and we have documented peer-reviewed evidence that it is possible to have the gene and not develop the illness then the illness is not correctly classified as a genetic illness. Some will argue that there is a genetic component but that is a red herring or an irrelevant argument.

Every state of health and illness has a genetic component. The issue is not if a gene is involved, genes are always involved. The issue is whether or not the presence of a gene is the determining factor or whether the expression of a gene is the determining factor.

If the illness is not present every time the gene is present then we know it is a gene-expression illness and not a gene-presence illness. Gene expression is determined by environment, gene expression is determined by lifestyle choice. Illnesses that involve gene expression are not genetic illnesses, they are lifestyle and/or environmental illnesses.

Can an illness be accurately defined as a genetic illness if it is possible to have the gene and not develop the illness?

Think about the fact that researchers have apparently recently discovered the "hangover gene". Now I can assure you that if such a gene did exist I got two of them. However, the reality is that I cannot blame my parents for my hangovers. Even if a "hangover gene" did exist, I can't get a hangover unless I drink poisonous alcohol. I could go my whole life with this gene and NEVER get a hangover. It is only if I get exposed to the stressor of poisonous alcohol that I get a hangover. Hangovers are lifestyle issues NOT genetic issues regardless of the presence of the gene. It is a gene expression issue NOT a gene presence issue. I bet you are seeing this very clearly when I talk about hangovers. It gets a bit more difficult when we talk about heart disease or cancer or obesity or diabetes even though the concept is identical. Thousands and thousands of women have lived long, full lives with the "breast cancer gene" and never developed breast cancer. The same is true for people with the "thrifty gene" that is involved in fat storage that they are trying to say is responsible for obesity – there are millions of people with this gene that live full lives and never become obese and tens of millions without it that do become obese.

Further, how can humans have a "hangover gene" if our genes were formed long before humans ever consumed alcohol? It can't be a hangover gene. How they name things has a great deal of influence on how we see things. They name things based on the assumption that genes are the cause.

Why would evolution keep a gene that caused cancer or diabetes, or obesity? Why would God implant those genes in humans? How can we explain the fact that these genes have always been present but that cancer, diabetes, obesity, heart disease and all the other chronic illnesses have been rapidly increasing over just a few decades?

I also like to point out that smoking only causes lung cancer in 50 percent of smokers. So should we call lung cancer a genetic illness or a lifestyle illness? Tobacco companies have argued that if smoking was the real cause of lung cancer then everyone who smoked would get lung cancer. By the way this is the EXACT defense tactic used by chemical companies, industrial polluters and pharmaceutical companies. The victims are forced to prove that the pollutant or drug caused their health issue. When the companies can show that there are some other humans who have been exposed to the same pollutants or drugs but have not developed the same cancer or other life destroying illness, the judge often has to rule in favor of the polluters or drug producers and prescription writers. I wish they knew the plant analogy! Those against smoking, ironically many of whom are blaming genes for every other type of cancer, would claim that those who smoke have a statistically significant greater chance of developing lung cancer so lung cancer must be a lifestyle disease caused by smoking. The fact that lung cancer is extremely rare in non-smokers is also important.

If the genes that cause cancer, heart disease, and all the other chronic illnesses have been present in the human genome all along why have the incidences of these illnesses been rising rapidly only over the past few decades?

Now imagine if you have years of exposure to thousands of different toxins and you develop cancer. How are you going to figure out which of these is to blame? Can you afford to sue every company that produced a toxin that you have been exposed to? Can you ever figure out what percent of your illness was caused by each individual toxin and thus what percent of your settlement should be paid by each individual company? If this topic interests you, especially if you are interested in how this topic relates to cancer, I highly recommend you read the book *The Secret War on Cancer* written by Dr. Devra Davis Ph.D., former researcher at the National Academy of Sciences and current Professor of Epidemiology and Director of the Center for Environmental Oncology at the University of Pittsburgh Cancer Institute.

Be prepared to be outraged at both those who make a living

while causing cancers and those who make a living developing treatments for cancer while they deliberately ignore the known environmental and lifestyle causes, the known preventions, and the lack of evidence and effectiveness of treatments. Just a completely gut wrenching look at how profit and paradigm drive traditional medicine and industry.

To be honest this entire debate is wasteful. Even conservative estimates are that less than five percent of chronic illness is attributable to genes.[42] Regardless of the exact small percentage, there are two important facts that simply cannot be denied. One, the vast majority of illness, spending, and deaths are attributable to lifestyle and thus preventable with lifestyle change. Two, lifestyle is the most significant factor determining the quality and quantity of life for at least 95% of the population and is a very significant factor determining quality of life in 100% of the population.

Regardless of what genes you have, what is the thing that determines whether or not you will express your genetic potential for health and vitality? How many people have you met that are expressing their full potential?

The important thing to always keep in mind is that genetic illnesses are not the chronic illnesses that are killing 80 percent of industrial humans or bankrupting individuals, companies, and governments. Most importantly, it is these preventable, chronic lifestyle illnesses that take up all the resources and divert them away from finding ways to help the unfortunate few that actually do suffer with genetic illness.

Even more importantly, it is the lifestyle choices of all of us, regardless of our gene code, that determine whether or not we experience our potential. It is so tragic that people with genetic illnesses suffer so needlessly from the addition of lifestyle illness because their lifestyle choices are so poor. Everyone benefits from healthy lifestyle choices and everyone suffers from unhealthy lifestyle choices. This is the take home point. A person with Down's Syndrome has a better life if they make healthy lifestyle choices. A person without Down's Syndrome has a better life if they make healthy lifestyle choices.

EVERY human, every member of every species, has a better life if they have a healthier environment. It's not complicated and it is not debatable.

Now, if you live in a stressor filled environment, if you have chronic toxicity and deficiency, your cells are going to go into a state of adaptation because they are genetically programmed to strive for survival. Let's remind ourselves one more time. If we are at a state of 7 out of 10 on the cell function and homeostasis scale what is the only way we can get more well or less sick? We must move towards 10. Is there any other way to make a human being or any other living creature more healthy or less sick other than improving the function of their cells? NO. So, healing and health are about improving cell function. There is no other way.

Remember that the most important things we can do in order to take control of our health is to answer the two most important questions about health accurately and to then take action based on those answers.

The first question we must answer is why we are sick. Only when we can accurately answer this question can we correctly answer the second important question. How do we get and stay well?

If we are sick because our cells are in a state of adaptation what is the only way to get healthier?

Essentially what we are asking is why our cells move into a state of adaptation or stress physiology. What stressors are forcing our cells into a state of stress and illness and what are the consequences of entering into and staying in these states of adaptation or stress?

Stressors: Why We Get Sick

Let's do a quick review. We now understand that health is validly defined in terms of states of cell function. We now also understand that sickness is validly defined as unsustainable adaptive cell function. We also understand that the reason cells enter a state of adaptation, a state of unhealthy cell function, a state of stress, is due to exposure to environmental or lifestyle stressors (toxicity and deficiency).

Understanding the role of chronic stressors and their chronic effects on physiology is the foundation of understanding chronic health and illness.

Hans Selye, who was a very famous Canadian researcher in the mid twentieth century, was one of the pioneering researchers regarding the cell function, health, and illness effects of chronic exposure to stressors. What Hans Selye discovered was that our body responds to virtually any stressor in the same way - at least initially. What this means is that our cells are stressed, are forced into a state of adaptation, by all toxicities and deficiencies, by all environmental stimuli that our nervous systems and genes identify as stressors. Hans Selye discovered that cells, and the organisms they form, go through a series of predictable stages when exposed to chronic stressors. The first stage is alarm or fight or flight. The individual cells, and the ecosystem or organism they make up, detect the stressor and change genetic expression in order to enter a state of alarm, a state of fear and protection, a state of survival physiology.

What happens to our state of cell function and overall health if we remain in a chronically stressful environment?

The next stage is adaptation. There is a deliberate and intelligent change in physiology that is aimed at surviving or, if possible, adapting to the threat imposed by the stressor – again this is based on genetic expression. The third stage is fatigue. If the exposure to the stressor is chronic the cells and/or entire organism expend so much energy dealing with this stressor that they become fatigued and weak and unable to deal with any other challenges. The last stage is death. If the chronic stressor remains it eventually completely exhausts our resources for survival and we die. This is a very accurate description of the stages of chronic illness. Chronic illness is the result of chronic stressors.[43]

Recently researchers like Schulkin, McEwan, Sterling, and Seaman have developed a more current model that explains the physiological cost of chronic adaptation to stressors. They have coined the term allostasis to describe the adaptive states of physiology that the body or human ecosystem enters into in response to environmental stressors. Allostatic load is the term used to describe the long term cost, or load, or tax that sustaining these adaptive states places on our bodies or ecosystems. The model clearly shows how these states do not represent genetic error or inherent cell pathology but are instead the result of the environment, the result of intelligent genetic expression changes in order to survive stressful environments.

These concepts, along with the concept of epigenetics, are not only explanatory in terms of how the environment is the root cause of chronic illness, but also why the Sickness & Treatment Paradigm is so ineffective and must be replaced by the Wellness & Prevention Paradigm.

Schulkin has recently edited a book titled 'Allostasis, Homeostasis, and the Costs of Physiological Adaptation' which I highly recommend for those of you more interested in the subject. There are also many references cited in the bibliography of this book.

The Rocks in our Backpack Stressor Analogy

The analogy I like to use to explain that chronic illness is the result of chronic stressors and chronic allostatic load is what I call my Rocks in our Backpack Stressor Analogy.

Imagine that you are born into a swimming pool wearing water wings and a backpack. Water wings are those little inflatable bands you wear around your arms to keep you afloat.

Imagine yourself in a swimming pool with water wings around your arms and a backpack on. Now it seems to be fairly well accepted that the human species has a genetically determined lifespan of around 120 years. In this analogy what this means is that you can think of being born into a swimming pool with a backpack on, with the water wings on, and those water wings have a very slow leak. This very slow leak means that the air will run out of those water wings in about 120 years. That's your species specific genetically determined lifespan potential. So if you are born into that pool, and there is no chronic stressors, you are just going to happily float around in there, and you are going to get your 120 years out of life.

What is the genetically determined lifespan for the human species? Why don't we all reach this?

Now, in this analogy, any form of stressor in your life, any toxicity or deficiency, any allostatic load, represents a rock in your backpack. Any form of stress in your life is a rock in that backpack. Now, what happens is when you get that rock in your backpack, a couple of things that are very important occur every single time. The first thing is that you sink a little bit lower in that water. What does that do to the pressure on your water wings? It increases it. What does that do to the rate of air leakage? It increases it. So what does this do to your rate of aging? It increases it. It means you are going to have less time on the planet.

This is exactly what chronic stress or allostatic load does to your rate of cell division. Stress increases the rate of cell division and thus decreases your lifespan. Stress also causes damage to your DNA and decreases your ability to repair it.[44]

The other thing that happens is when you sink a little lower in the water, because you've got that rock or that stress load in your backpack weighing you down, day-to-day life becomes a little bit more of a struggle. You've got to work a little bit harder to keep your nose above water.

Chronic stress or allostatic load increases the metabolic cost of daily survival and stress causes a decrease in your quality of life – stressors are emotionally stressful as well as physically stressful.

How does exposure to chronic stressors affect quality and quantity of life?

So two things always happen when we expose ourselves to chronic environmental stressors, when we put rocks in our backpack, when we have allostatic load. The first thing is that we shorten our lifespan. Our cells start to divide quicker. We have more cell damage, and we actually have less lifespan. But more importantly, the quality of our life also decreases, and day to day life becomes more of a struggle. And what I'll tell you is that it does not matter what drug or surgery you get when you're in that pool with that rock in your backpack. The only thing that matters is getting the rock out of the backpack, decreasing your allostatic load.

What I want you to learn from this is book is to take control over what rocks go in and what rocks you're going to take out, and to understand that simply treating the effects of those rocks in your backpack, such as changes in blood pressure or changes in cholesterol, will never address the cause of the issue and never return you to a state of balance and health.

Unless we address the cause, we have no hope. And the cause is not bad genes, bad cells, or bad luck. The cause is bad lifestyle choices that put rocks in our backpack or a stress load (allostatic load) on our physiology.

The Sickness & Treatment Paradigm espouses the belief that the changes in your cell function, your quality of life, and your lifespan as you sink in the pool are caused by bad genes or dysfunctioning cells. The Wellness & Prevention Paradigm espouses the belief that these changes are caused by the rocks or the stressors you put in your backpack from your environment and from your lifestyle choices. The Sickness & Treatment Paradigm is about giving you drugs and surgery to address the EFFECTS of the rocks in your backpack. The Wellness & Prevention Paradigm is about removing those rocks or stressors and teaching you how to avoid them. When it comes to chronic illness the research is clear, the Wellness & Prevention Paradigm is correct.

Really think about how often you are under chronic stress and have rocks in your backpack. My goal is to help you get the rocks out, not to make you feel better with the rocks in. That's the fundamental difference between traditional medicine and what I'm trying to teach you. Think about it. Do drugs and surgery take rocks out of your backpack and result in decreased allostatic load or healthier cell function? This is an incredibly important question, because the truth is that I will never be so ridiculous or unscientific to suggest that there is never an appropriate time to take a drug or have surgery. What I will always say, and will insist that you must understand, is that there is never an appropriate time to take a drug if you believe it is going to create more health for you or address the cause of your chronic illness. Drugs can treat your sickness and symptoms but they cannot make you well.

Do drugs or surgery remove the chronic stressors from your environment or lifestyle?

Again an important point to consider is that the only viable solution to a health issue caused by chronic stressors is to remove the stressor from the human or to remove the human from the stressful environment. Simply taking a drug to treat the adaptive effects of the stressor is not logical. We will come back to this point over and over again. It is just so important.

Let me give you a quick lesson regarding chronic stressors and how your body intelligently attempts to adapt and survive. Let me tell you a little bit about what chronic stress does to you, so that you can really understand the effects and thus make an intelligent decision about what solution to pursue when you find yourself in the stage of adaptation or fatigue.

The Causes of Illness and the Requirements for Health are Species Specific

Before we learn about the effects of chronic stressors we need to define what a chronic stressor is.

Stressors that cause the genetic expression of adaptive physiology, or fatigue or illness physiology are species-specific. In other words, what might be stressful for a human animal might in fact be required by another animal species, like a panda bear or a sloth.

What determines whether or not an environmental stimuli is a stressor? What determines whether or not we enter a state of alarm or adaptation?

What determines which species we belong to is gene code. Each species has a unique gene code. Animals of the same species can mate and produce offspring because their gene codes, or recipes for life, or blueprints for life, are similar enough that when they mate and each contribute half the required DNA to form a zygote these two halves of genetic material are so similar that they can fit together and produce viable offspring (kind of takes the romance out of it doesn't it). As genes contain the recipe of life, if the recipes from the parents are not similar enough then the offspring, or the bun cooked up in the oven, is not viable. If you have one parent donating the genetic recipe for a bun and the other a meatloaf, they will not form a bun-loaf, and even if they did it would not be viable. If you have a giraffe mate with a horse the DNA, the gene codes, the recipes of life, are too different to create a viable life.

It is our gene code that determines what type of environment we need to live in and it is the environment we live in that determines how we will express the genes we have.

Genes have been shaped by the environment over millennia and the recipes that are in those genes are specific to each species and specific to the environment that was present when the genome for that species was formed or evolved, or, if you prefer, created. For example, the human genome as it now stands was formed about 10-20,000 years ago and thus we are genetically best suited, and thus genetically require, an environment and lifestyle we had 10,000 years ago.

In other words, we have hunter-gatherer genes but we now live in an industrial environment. This mismatch, this incongruity between our genetic requirements or our genetic code and our environment, is at the root of all chronic illness. We will come back to this again and again.

Each species requires the ingredients from the environment specific to the unique recipes of that species. It is your genes that determine what you require in terms of sufficient ingredients and it is your genes that determine what things will be toxic to you. The required ingredients for your genetic recipe (or the required building materials for your genetic blueprint if you prefer) and what environmental stimuli will be toxic, are determined by your gene code. Stressors and required ingredients are species specific. A stressor can thus be defined as exposure to something that is toxic or a deficiency of something that is required for cell function. Toxicity and deficiency, as you have learned, are the two categories that all stressors can be divided into.

What determines what ingredients or raw materials we require from the environment? What determines what is defined as sufficient or deficient?

Why is this important to know? It is important to know so that you can understand the importance of making genetically congruent lifestyle choices. It is important to know so that you can understand what the determining factor is in identifying what lifestyle choices are healthy and what lifestyle choices are unhealthy.

Healthy choices are genetically congruent choices, healthy choices are those choices that supply the right ingredients in the right amounts and healthy choices are those choices that avoid toxic stressors.

Healthy choices are sufficient and pure. Unhealthy choices are deficient and toxic and all this is based on your species specific genetic requirements.

Lack of this understanding is why health can be so confusing and why there is so much misinformation regarding nutrition, exercise, and psychosocial factors. The reason there are so many different 'diets' and 'diet' books and so many different "exercise plans" and so many different "self help" books is because nobody has been asking the right questions. None have asked or answered the right questions, so none have come up with the right answers.

What we must do is determine what constitutes genetically congruent nutrition for the human species, what constitutes genetically congruent movement and energy expenditure patterns for the human species, and what constitutes genetically congruent intra and interpersonal communication and relationship patterns for the human species.

We must determine what constitutes purity and sufficiency and toxicity and deficiency for the human species. I have asked and endeavored to answer these exact questions in my three text series: *The Innate Diet, Innate Physical Fitness*, and the *Innate State of Mind* (these texts are very research heavy and written specifically as texts for the post-graduate wellness lifestyle certification program that I teach. I am writing a book for the laypublic that covers this material).

What defines a healthy lifestyle choice?

Interestingly I have noticed a significant increase in the number of Sickness & Treatment Paradigm practitioners attending my lay lectures and have also noticed, as you will see from the quoted research in later chapters, a significant increase in discussion of lifestyle and gene expression or epigenetics and allostatic load in the peer-reviewed literature. In fact there is now a peer-reviewed journal titled the *American Journal of Lifestyle Medicine*.

The articles are not always written within the Wellness & Prevention Paradigm but the journal as a whole is leaps and bounds further toward this (and further away from the Sickness & Treatment Paradigm) than 99.9 percent of all the other available literature. I applaud the editorial board for their efforts and I am a paid subscriber.

There is also a journal titled *Epigenetics* and as previously mentioned the fabulous book *Allostasis, Homeostasis, and the Cost of Physiological Adaptation* that represent very significant, although not complete, paradigm shifts. As always it will take the mainstream clinical education and delivery systems one or more decades to shift and even this will only occur if they can remove the economic and educational influence (really monopoly) of the pharmaceutical companies whose power and profits depend on the perpetuation of the Sickness & Treatment Paradigm.

The Causes of Illness and the Requirements for Health are Species Wide

The next thing that is very important to understand is that toxicity and deficiency and purity and sufficiency are species wide. In other words, stressors that cause the genetic expression of adaptation, fatigue, death - and the required ingredients or raw materials for the expression of health - are species wide. This is sometimes hard to grasp, especially for health care practitioners who are trained and indoctrinated in the belief system that the causes of illness and their treatments are disease specific or individual specific and thus require specific treatments for specific diagnoses.

The truth is that the causes of illness and the sources of healing are not individual, they are species wide, especially when it comes to chronic illness.

Is what constitutes purity and sufficiency and/or toxicity and deficiency different for each individual member of a species?

The truth is that humans are so genetically similar that we simply have to have virtually identical requirements in terms of what is genetically congruent or what ingredients we need for our genetic recipes of life.

Let's move away from human animals for a second because your bias is so strong when it comes to humans. Think back to the great lake analogy or go back and reread it. Or just for a moment ask yourself what other animal species has individual rather than species wide requirements in terms of nutrition, exercise and energy expenditure, or psychosocial patterns. Does one giraffe require different food types than the next? Does one polar bear require different food types than the next? Does one giraffe or polar bear require different exercise and energy expenditure patterns or different psychosocial patterns than the next? Of course not. So why would human animals? They wouldn't.

The fact is that humans all require the same things in terms of essential nutrients, exercise, and positive intra and interpersonal relationships. Similarly, things that are stressors for one human are virtually always stressors for all humans - the exceptions to this are emotional stressors and some allergies. The fact is that you don't need to add or remove anything from your life that should not be added or removed from everyone else's. Humans are no different than any other species when it comes to this issue. Anyone who is trying to convince you otherwise is trying to take advantage of you or take your money.

Now sharing the truth might cost me some money in terms of selling you the next health fad but the lies that are currently believed are costing millions of lives and hundreds of billions of dollars – per year! I'm willing to give up the health fad revenue to save lives and save healthcare. I wish this was a more commonly held point of view.

Does every individual giraffe or polar bear or hippopotamus have different requirements in terms of eating, moving, thinking, and interacting? Does every individual human?

Back to stressors or rocks in your backpack or allostatic load and the effects chronic stressors have on our physiology and our health. All stressors can be categorized into toxicity and deficiency. Being exposed to toxins or not getting sufficient amounts of the raw materials or ingredients your genetic blueprint or recipe requires is stressful and represents a rock in your backpack.

So if you eat a bad meal, that's a stressor, a rock in your backpack. If you don't eat a good meal, that's a stressor, a rock in your backpack. If you don't exercise, that's a stressor, another rock in your backpack. If you have bad posture, or your spine or other joints have scar tissue from trauma or sedentary living and cannot move properly, that's a stressor, another rock in your backpack. If you think negative thoughts about yourself or others, that's a stressor, another rock in your backpack. If you don't think enough positive thoughts about yourself or others, that's a stressor, another rock in your backpack. If you don't feel safe and loved and important in your social networks or if you don't have social networks, that's a stressor, another rock in your backpack. If you have toxins in your environment and pollutants, that's a stressor, another rock in your backpack.

Just stop for a moment and think about how many rocks you put in your backpack last week. Think how many you have put in throughout your lifetime. Rocks bio-accumulate and your backpack gets heavier and heavier and you sink lower and lower in the water and your life becomes more and more of a struggle and you feel more and more tired and you get fatigued and maybe even depressed or anxious. You most likely blame all this on getting older or having bad genes. At this point you usually go to the doctor and get a pill.

The pill is almost always nothing more than another rock in your backpack that simply makes you feel a little better or at least numbs you a little bit regarding the effects of all the other rocks in your backpack. And so goes the story of ever-increasing chronic illness and ever-increasing prescriptions and ever-increasing costs and ever-decreasing health.

The Iceberg Analogy: Buying Time to Change our Environment

Something that is very important to understand is that going into acute states of adaptation, although not healthy, is very intelligent. The goal of your stressor response system, your environmental stressor survival response, is not to make you well. The sole goal of this system is to buy you some survival time while you are in the presence of acute environmental threats or stressors (to help you keep your head above water while you find a way to get the rock out of your backpack).

The goal is not to buy some survival time for healing. The goal is to buy you some survival time as you look for a way to change your environment, a way to remove yourself from the stressor in the environment, or to remove the stressor from your environment.

This system is very willing to create unhealthy physiology if it is capable of increasing your chance of survival. Health is irrelevant if you don't survive. You can recover from a shift away from health, you cannot recover from death.

If you are on an iceberg what is your body's response, what happens to your physiology? You pool the blood away from your extremities and shift it to your organs and to your brain. Now the question you need to ask is whether this is an act of stupidity or an act of intelligence. You also need to ask if this represents health or sickness and if it represents pathological error or deliberate adaptive response.

The answer is that it represents sickness; just ask the big toe that is getting gangrene. However, it is anything but an act of stupidity, in fact, it is an act of extreme intelligence, not conscious intellect but innate genetic intelligence. It is also not pathological

What is the goal of the flight or fight response, of entering into a state of adaptation? Is this pathological or intelligent? Is it healthy or unhealthy?

error it is a very deliberate adaptive response. It's intelligent because it buys you time to survive on the iceberg. Why would your innate genetic intelligence deliberately create a state of physiology that causes sickness (gangrene)? This is the important question, this is the paradigm shifting question. There's only one reason your body will actually go into a state of sickness or catabolism or emergency breakdown for survival. It literally is an alarm response.

The innate genetic intelligence of your body is programmed to operate within a hierarchy of response choice that puts your survival as the top priority. In other words, your innate intelligence is willing to let the big toe die in order to save your organs and your brain because your organs and your brain are required for your survival and your big toe is not.

How is this intelligent, how does this increase our chance of survival? Again, this is absolutely key, this is paradigm shifting. What you need to understand is that, regardless of how intelligent your response is, regardless of whether or not you can increase survival time, there is a limit.

Is the survival response or adaptation response meant to be the solution to the stressor?

This response is NOT meant to be the solution. This response is meant to buy you some time to find the solution.

In our iceberg example this response is meant to buy you enough time to get off the iceberg, TO BUY YOU TIME TO CHANGE YOUR ENVIRONMENT. That's the only reason your body is every going into that stress response. It's to buy you enough time to get off the iceberg or to stop eating junk food. It's to buy you enough time to get off the couch. It's to buy you enough time to start looking in the mirror and telling yourself how great you are, and how important you are, and how you love yourself, and love your kids. It's to buy you enough time to get the rocks out of your backpack. That's why your body goes into that state of stress, to buy you time to get your environment right, to get away from the tiger.

The problem is that the traditional medical view, based on the Sickness & Treatment Paradigm, is that these states of stress represent pathological error and thus must be corrected with prescription drugs or surgery.

It doesn't matter what drug you take on the iceberg, if you don't get off of the iceberg, it's over. You could develop a drug to stop the pooling of the blood to your organs and to your brain and I'm sure you could develop a surgery to shunt blood to your big toe. You could even do a randomized controlled trial that would provide evidence that these interventions could stop or treat gangrene of the toe. In the meantime the person is still on the iceberg and they are still dying. They will just die without gangrene. Further, they will, in all likelihood, continue to ignore the fact they are on the iceberg because they don't even have the gangrene as a huge wake up call to let them know they are in trouble.

The Sickness & Treatment Paradigm ignores the iceberg, considers the changes in physiology associated with living on that iceberg pathological error, and focuses on treating the effects of being on the iceberg with drugs and surgery.

The Wellness & Prevention Paradigm focuses on the iceberg, considers the changes in physiology associated with living on that iceberg as deliberate and intelligent and as an indicator that the environment is pathological, and intervenes with advice and empowerment about how to change that environment or move to a more suitable one.

Does the traditional medical view see states of adaptation as intelligent or as pathological?

Chapter 6
How Chronic Stress Becomes Chronic Illness: The Physiology of Chronic Adaptation

"Every stress leaves an indelible scar, and the organism pays for its survival after a stressful situation by becoming a little older."

Dr. Hans Selye

Now that we have a basic understanding of the concepts of stressors, adaptive physiology and illness we can now explore the causal relationship between chronic stressors and chronic illness. We have some more important questions to ask and answer. What happens when humans live in a chronically stressful environment, when we choose to chronically eat, move, think, and interact in genetically incongruent ways? What changes in physiology and health take place when humans are under chronic stress, when we have chronic toxicity and/or deficiency? As Hans Selye taught us, the changes that take place are predictable and consistent. We enter a state of physiological adaptation, followed by a state of fatigue, and, finally, if we fail to remove the stressors from our environment, or move to a less stressful environment, we die. As we move along this path we develop chronic illness. Chronic illness is the direct result of chronic exposure to environmental or lifestyle stressors.

Remember, your state of physiology and your state of cell function are the genetic expression of your environment. Your state of health is the genetic expression of your past and present environments.

To fully understand this we need to first understand that the chronic release of stress hormones is due to chronic exposure to stressful environmental stimuli. I think we get this point by now. The next thing we need to understand is the effect of chronically increased stress hormones; we need to understand the chronic physiological and health changes associated with chronically elevated stress hormones and chronically elevated allostatic load. There are two main categories of stress hormones that get deliberately and intelligently elevated in response to chronic stress. These two types of hormones are catecholamines (adrenaline and noradrenaline or epinephrine and norepinephrine) and cortisol.

Let's start with a broad overview of what these hormones do. The first thing that happens is that stress hormones increase heart rate, cardiac output, blood pressure, and blood flow to parts of the body and brain for flight or fight (fear and protection) and decrease blood flow to parts of the body and brain for healing, growth, and repair (relaxation and exploration). Stress hormones literally down regulate all the processes to do with anabolism or growth and up regulate all the processes to do with catabolism or body breakdown for emergency response.

Is it possible to develop chronic illness without being chronically exposed to environmental or lifestyle stressors?

Stress hormones put you into a state of alarm to maximize your survival by maximizing your chance to change your environment (fight) or move to a more suitable environment (flight).

Let's now look at some specific physiological effects of stress hormones. As you wind your way through this information always keep in mind how appropriate and intelligent these adaptations are in terms of increasing your chance of survival. Once you have finished going through all these adaptations ask yourself what the long term health effects of these adaptations would be if they were chronically sustained.

Remember, chronically sustaining these changes does NOT represent pathology, it represents necessary, appropriate, and intelligent responses to chronic stressors, to chronic rocks in your backpack.

The following summary of the physiological changes associated with the alarm or stress response and how sustaining these responses leads to states of adaptation and fatigue (allostatic load) are excerpted from two of my previous books – 'Innate Physical Fitness' and 'The Innate State of Mind'. Although there are some physiological terms there is nothing that you will not understand. Focus on seeing the big picture and do not concern yourself with memorizing every detail. You can always reread the section or write out some flow charts at a later time if you choose to commit the material to memory. For now just seek to understand the big picture of how chronic stressful or genetically incongruent or pathological lifestyle choices elicit intelligent physiological adaptations that represent an allostatic load and can ultimately lead to fatigue, chronic illness, and death.

The first thing to occur is that your brain and nervous system detect a threat or a stressor (i.e. a tiger leaping at you or some other form of toxicity or deficiency).

Your brain and nervous system send signals to the cell bodies of the sympathetic nervous system located in the intermediolateral tract (IML) of your spinal cord where the stress response or fight or flight response is initiated. The sympathetic system directly influences visceral (organ) function via neuronal control of these organs. All fear and protection or fight or flight functions required to survive the threat are up regulated (i.e. heart rate and blood pressure, increased blood sugar etc) and all anabolic or growth and repair activities are down regulated (i.e. growth hormone, immunity, digestion, sex drive). You don't need growth and repair for survival during an attack from a tiger so this represents a very intelligent adaptation or shift in physiology to meet the environmental demand.

Is the immune system important during an acute threat of attack?

Stress hormones, particularly cortisol, down-regulate your cell-mediated immune system.[45] Your immune system is very metabolically expensive. This is why you get tired when you have a cold or a flu. You get tired because you have to boost up your immune system, and that takes a lot of energy, a lot of glucose, and it's very tiring. So why would your body prioritize energy toward operating your immune system if the priority is to escape from a tiger? It wouldn't. Think about it, would you like to have your white blood cells in charge of protecting you from the tiger attack? So your immune system is basically useless to you, unless or until you survive the attack and are wounded, then your immune system becomes very important.

The sympathetic system (IML) sends a message directly to your adrenal glands (uniquely, when sending a message to the adrenal glands the sympathetic system does not synapse at the sympathetic chain ganglia – this is because we need to get the information to the adrenal glands RIGHT NOW). Of course by this time your brain is also sending messages to the adrenal glands via the hypothalamic - pituitary - adrenal axis.

The adrenals produce catecholamines (adrenaline/ noradrenaline – epinephrine/norepinephrine) from the medulla and glucocorticoid (cortisol) from the cortex.[46] Catecholamines act on the heart to sustain increased cardiac output (heart rate and stroke volume) – this, along with vasoconstriction from sympathetic system output, serves to increase blood pressure – this allows rapid delivery of stress response hormones and energy substrates. The stress response also results in the release of plasmin and other clotting factors into the blood in preparation for a possible wound.[47]

Catecholamines stimulate the amygdala (stress and anxiety center) in the brain so that emotional/anxiety memories dominate during stress (so we remember to look for the tiger next time we are at the watering hole).[48]

Why are more clotting factors released into the bloodstream during the alarm response?

Catecholamines inhibit factual learning, working memory and the ability to focus attention at a part of the brain called the hippocampus (you don't need to be able to learn history or memorize a poem while running from a tiger).

The amygdala releases a hormone called corticotropin releasing hormone CRH (CRF) which activates another part of the stress pathway in the brain called the locus ceruleus which releases noradrenaline that acts on emotional centers and learning centers in the brain (areas for logical behaviour and short term memory get inhibited; centers for emotional learning and instinctual behaviour get stimulated). This is innately intelligent as it allows the best chance to survive via flight or fight.[49]

Release of noradrenaline during the stress response causes an increased sensitivity of the sensory systems (this improves chances of detecting a method of survival during fight/flight). However, this means our concentration is easily distracted and this is why when we are stressed out we cannot focus our attention very well. As Michael Meaney Ph.D. describes it, "Stress sharpens the signal detection system at the cost of concentration."[50] When we are stressed we become very easily distracted and have trouble learning new information (sounds like ADHD and adult burnout doesn't it?). Haven't you noticed when people are stressed out that they become kind of twitchy and irritable? They are looking all around, but they're not really good at focusing. This is why it is rarely successful to phone your spouse when they are stressed out in traffic on the way home and give them a list of things to pick up at the store. If you are lucky they come home with two, the first and the last on the list, and then they're under even more stress because they forgot the stuff. This is also why some students don't perform well on tests even though they know the material so well in class or during studying. If they get stressed out during the exam they just don't concentrate well or recall information very well. Their brains are searching for an escape route instead of answers.

Can humans stimulate or inhibit their own adaptation responses with conscious thoughts?

Studies show that chronic stress physiology can lead to chronic changes in cognition - under chronic stress cells in the hippocampus actually shrink and can die.[51] Interestingly research also shows that chronic movement stimulation or exercise results in an increase in the size and number of hippocampal cells; exercise actually directly increases and/or helps restore the ability to learn and remember and can significantly decrease (by up to 70 percent) the incidence of Parkinson's and dementia.[52, 53] Exercise actually counteracts the effects of stress, exercise increases your adaptability and your ability to cope with stress.

The locus ceruleus also acts on another part of the brain stress pathway called the hypothalamus and initiates the hypothalamic-pituitary-adrenal axis which leads to increased release of the stress hormones (catecholamines and cortisol) which is needed to maintain the alarm response and/or adaptive response.

An interesting and important point to know is that humans, as conscious animals, have the ability to inhibit or stimulate these pathways with our thoughts and perceptions.

Positive thoughts and emotions initiated in the left prefrontal cortex can inhibit the stress response by releasing GABA (an inhibitory neurotransmitter) at the amygdala. In other words we, as humans, can consciously choose to react differently to stimuli and significantly lower our own emotional stress levels – and thus our allostatic load levels – take rocks out of our backpacks – by choosing to focus on things like gratitude and solutions rather than resentment and problems.[54]

Humans can also stimulate the stress response by consciously thinking about a stressful past event (dwelling on the loss of our job, a bad test score, or a bad hair day) or anticipating a future stressful event (sitting in a dentist waiting room before a root canal, thinking about having to tell your spouse you smashed the car). In fact, during periods of chronic stress it becomes easier to dwell on the negative aspects of life.

We actually get better at anything we repeatedly do or practice; this includes stressful, anxious, or depressing thoughts. When we make a lot of neural connections or synapses along these negative or stressful pathways the glass is more easily seen as half empty. We are more sensitive and over-reactive because these pathways are literally sensitized. Sound familiar? The good news is that we can also become sensitized along the glass half full pathways.

Can chronic stressors and chronic adaptation to chronic stressors change our moods and our general outlook on life?

The research is very clear, a good attitude makes us healthier and a bad attitude makes us sicker.[55] We can practice and develop synapses and habits along good or bad pathways – which are you choosing to practice and develop?

The stress response, because it activates the brain systems that concentrate on threat and anxiety and fires the sympathetic or fight or flight nervous system, also results in a decreased ability to sleep. This is very significant because research shows that shortening even one night's sleep by 4 hours causes significant increase in stress hormone release. You can see that this can become a self perpetuating cycle.[56]

Under normal conditions SEROTONIN is released to inhibit the activity of the noradrenergic cells of the locus ceruleus that lead to anxiety and depression. Serotonin is produced to get us back to balance and homeostasis after we've fired off the stress pathways. HOWEVER, under chronic stress (chronically living in a genetically incongruent environment, chronic allostatic load/rocks in the backpack) serotonin production cannot keep up and the result is that serotonin levels drop – we use up all our serotonin for anti-anxiety and we don't have any left over to help us feel good.

The result of this combination of increased noradrenaline and decreased serotonin levels is that people get depressed, feel irritable, tired, listless, have problems sleeping, get tension headaches, have decreased sex drive, get lowered growth hormone levels, and get changes in appetite and gain weight – they crave sugar and fat!

Fat and sugar are the main ingredients for our stress hormones, so when we are under stress we actually require more fats and sugars. Sound familiar, do you have such cravings when you are stressed out, do you seek 'comfort foods' when you are stressed?

Why do we crave fatty, sugary "comfort' foods when we are under stress?

Of course we are genetically designed to derive our fat and sugar from fruits and vegetables, nuts and seeds, and wild game meat like our ancestors did. Industrial humans now consume processed non-fiber carbohydrates in the form of refined sugar and high fructose corn syrup and fats in the form of trans fats or hydrogenated fats in foods filled with chemical colors and preservatives. This just adds rocks to our backpack as we get 'comfortable' from eating these toxic, deficient foods and the cycle gets perpetuated. Add in the insulin resistance from chronic high blood glucose levels and chronic high insulin levels leading to type II diabetes and you get syndrome X or burnout or chronic fatigue and increased chance of cancer and heart disease and every other chronic illness.[57]

In any case, when you fire off your anxiety and your stress responses in your body, there are two main ways to get back to homeostasis: serotonin or exercise. Exercise actually stimulates movement-pleasure pathways that produce the brain and hormonal patterns for feeling better.

The take home point is that the way to get back to "normal" is to move to a "normal" environment. A "normal" environment for a human includes eating, moving, and thinking well, it includes eating, moving, thinking, and interacting in genetically congruent ways. "Normal" does not include psychotropic drugs while we sit on the couch eating junk food to try and feel better.

Cortisol and catecholamines also epigenetically downregulate

"In Spark, I'll demonstrate how and why physical activity is crucial to the way we think and feel. I'll explain the science of how exercise cues the building blocks of the brain; how it affects mood, anxiety, and attention; how it guards against stress and reverses some of the effects of aging in the brain."

Ratey, John. (2008) Spark: The Revolutionary New Science of Exercise and the Brain. Little, Brown and Company, New York, New York, USA.

insulin receptors. These are the receptors that take the blood sugar out of our bloodstream, so this is actually down-regulated except at those areas such as skeletal muscle that need the glucose for energy for fight or flight.[58] We do this because we don't want to be storing blood sugar if we are being chased by a tiger, we want to be utilizing that sugar for energy. In an acute stress response this is of course logical because you don't want to be anabolic and store the blood sugar you need for energy for flight or flight but if this becomes chronic it leads to type II diabetes, heart disease, obesity, cancers, and a plethora of other chronic conditions.

Is it possible that the adaptations that increase our survival under acute threat can, if sustained, lead to chronic illness?

The increase in blood glucose leads to more insulin production but the receptors are resistant so glucose levels stay high and the cycle continues until the pancreas can no longer keep up. It is also important to understand that insulin is a very powerful stimulator of the sympathetic nervous system when it is present in high levels so this leads to further increases in stress hormone levels.

Insulin resistance has also been linked to increased excretion of Ca++ in the urine and less IGF (insulin-like growth factor) stimulation of bone growth which can lead to osteoporosis. In addition insulin resistance lowers Mg++ levels. Mg++ is required for muscle relaxation so blood vessels constrict even more leading to further increases in blood pressure (vasoconstriction).

Thyroid hormones also get converted or activated in the liver. However, if you are insulin resistant this does not happen as it is supposed to. Growth hormone also gets activated at the liver via the insulin-like growth factors or somatomedins produced in the liver.

Again, this does not occur properly if the liver is insulin resistant. So you are aware, liver is the first tissue that becomes resistant to insulin, it is the most vulnerable.

Catecholamines also cause the liberation of free fatty acids (from selected fat stores) into the blood so that they can be used for gluconeogenesis (to make glucose) to provide necessary energy substrate for fight or flight – free fatty acids and glycerol can be used to form glucose via gluconeogenesis in the kreb's cycle. During periods of stress we selectively store excess fat centripetally (hips to thighs). Sound familiar? Look in the mirror or look at the waist-hip ratio of 100 people as they walk past you at a mall or airport. I'm sure you are aware that centripetal obesity is highly associated with diabetes, heart disease and virtually every other chronic illness including cancer. This is not because centripetal obesity is the cause of these other illnesses, it is because the physiological adaptation (and fatigue) that leads to centripetal obesity also leads to chronic illness.

Why is centripetal obesity associated with so many chronic illnesses?

Cortisol acts on the liver and causes the breakdown of glycogen stores into glucose to increase blood glucose levels in order to provide energy substrate for fight or flight. Cortisol also causes the breakdown of protein stores for gluconeogenesis (glucogenic amino acids are used to form glucose in gluconeogenic pathways of kreb's cycle).

Cortisol also acts at the liver and epigenetically downregulates the genetic expression of HDL cholesterol production and also epigenetically downregulates the number of receptors for LDL cholesterol. The net effect of this is that less HDL cholesterol gets produced and released into the bloodstream and less LDL gets taken out of bloodstream.[59]

But doesn't this mean that we have less 'good' cholesterol and more 'bad' cholesterol? Is this not evidence that the genes are bad or that the cells are operating incorrectly? Of course not. There is no such thing as good or bad cholesterol, only appropriate or inappropriate cholesterol levels. Appropriate to what is the most important question. Appropriate to the environmental demand is the answer. The adaptive (not pathological) changes in cholesterol levels are totally necessary during stress because cholesterol is important as a precursor for the steroid based hormones. Cholesterol is also used in healing wounds that might occur during fight or flight and is also very important in mood regulation after the threat (research shows that some become depressed and even suicidal when on cholesterol lowering drugs).[60]

Now if you are comparing cholesterol levels (or any other levels) to an artificially derived "appropriate level" you would consider them high. The problem is that the Sickness & Treatment Paradigm sets "appropriate" as those levels appropriate in a relaxed or homeostatic environment. They then consider any changes from these levels as pathological and "treat" what they consider as a genetic or cellular error with drugs in an attempt to bring the level back to "appropriate".

The error they are making is that the environment is not relaxed, it is stressful, and the adaptive responses to this stressful environment are appropriate and intelligent not pathological. Even worse, the drug companies and the medical researchers they employ just keep working harder and harder to have these "appropriate" or "healthy" levels set lower and lower so they can get more and more people consuming their drugs. They literally spend billions of dollars on lobbying government and marketing directly to doctors and to the public.

How do medical "experts" or pharmaceutical companies decide what levels of cholesterol or blood pressure are appropriate and healthy?

Let me give a very brief insight into this. There are many books and articles written on the topic of unethical drug research and over prescribing medications but that is not what this book is about. However, I think it is highly relevant that, as you begin to view health and sickness through the Wellness & Prevention Paradigm and start to understand the real underlying reasons about why humans get chronic illness, you also get some insight into why the current Sickness & Treatment Paradigm can never be the solution. I also think it is useful to get some insight into the evidence regarding the concept of following the paradigm and the profit to understand the reasons why the current system is so stubbornly drug-centric.

In 2001 the National Cholesterol Education Program created new guidelines regarding what was to be considered "normal" levels of cholesterol. Overnight the number of Americans that were deemed to require cholesterol medication (statin drugs) jumped from 13 million to 36 million.[61]

The guidelines cited only six studies to support their new recommendations. Five of the six studies were not prevention studies; the one prevention study that was cited was NOT statistically significant.[62] In other words there was NO SCIENTIFICALLY VALID EVIDENCE to support the guidelines.

As Dr. John Abramson, clinical instructor at Harvard Medical School points out in his book, *Overdosed America: The Broken Promise of American Medicine*, "Eight of the nine members of the guidelines panel had financial ties to the makers of cholesterol lowering drugs."[63]

"Most of the people who have heart attacks don't have elevated cholesterol, and most of the people who have elevated cholesterol don't have heart attacks."

Dr. Jim Wright - Professor - Department of Pharmacology, Therapeutics and Medicine. University of British Columbia in Heart of the Matter, CBC Radio - Ideas http://www.cbc.ca/ideas/IDEAS-Catalog.pdf

Have you ever seen any valid evidence to indicate that high cholesterol is the cause of heart disease or is this just something you assumed based on "expert" opinion?

As more and more of this evidence has come to light the drug makers have had to change their cholesterol lowering drug ads; they now have small print that states that the drugs have not been shown to prevent heart disease. Yet these remain among the most commonly prescribed and most highly profitable drugs in the world!

I'm sure many of you are finding this hard to believe; it is just so contrary to the "expert" opinion you have been hearing. Perhaps you should ask yourself where your doctor gets the information she or he disseminates about cholesterol drugs. I highly recommend that you do not take my word as gospel on this topic or any other. I encourage you to read more on this topic. I suggest you start with Dr. Abramson's book or one of

"Importantly, the only significant overall effect of cholesterol-lowering intervention that has ever been shown is increased mortality."

Atrens, D.M. The questionable wisdom of a low-fat diet and cholesterol reduction. Soc. Sci Med. 1994 39 (3):433-47 the many others that have been written on the topic. You could also get the transcript from a FANTASTIC summary of the controversy regarding the lack of scientific data supporting the 'cholesterol as the cause of heart disease myth' via a series of interviews with world renowned scientific and clinical experts that aired on CBC radio entitled *The Heart of the Matter.* The link to order the transcript is http://www.cbc.ca/ideas/IDEAS-Catalog.pdf I prefer the peer-reviewed scientific literature, for those that are the same each of the above have an abundance of references – too many to list here.

Let's segue back to our discussion of the effects of stress hormones at the liver. One of the other effects of insulin resistant liver cells is that it causes a decrease in the production of sex hormone binding globulin (SHBG). When you are chronically under stress, when you have chronic rocks in your backpack or chronic allostatic load, you become insulin resistant and your liver produces less of what's called sex hormone binding globulin. The important thing about binding sex hormones is that sex hormones are very mitogenic meaning they stimulate a lot of rapid cell division. So if you look at the research what you will see is that a low level of sex hormone binding globulin (a higher level of circulating unbound sex hormone) is a strong predictor of site specific cancers. The reason for this is that the less sex hormone binding globulin you have, the more free sex hormone you have rushing around in your bloodstream. So the more unbound sex hormone you have, the more it can get to areas that it's not supposed to go to. If it's bound, it gets escorted and taken to the place where it's supposed to go. If it is unbound it can go anywhere and cause rapid cell division. Now, if you combine that with a down-regulated immune system, your chances of cancer under chronic stress or chronic allostatic load are significantly increased.

Since the big high carbohydrate, low fat diet push from the dietary "experts" have obesity rates increased or decreased?

The immune system is supposed to find cancer cells and kill them, but if you have a lot of insulin which is very mitogenic, a lot of blood sugar that down regulates your immune function and feeds these cancer cells because you're eating a high carb diet, and you've got low sex hormone binding globulin, what happens? Think about the women that went on hormone replacement therapy. What happened to the rates of breast cancer? They went up because they were adding free sex hormone and they were told to go on a high-carb, low fat diet which decreased their immune system function. So they became insulin resistant and then they had less sex hormone binding globulin being produced and they got rapid cell division in breast tissue.

By the way, exercise decreases insulin resistance, increases sex hormone binding globulin levels and decreases the rate of site specific cancers - SIGNIFICANTLY.

As a quick side note an increased carbohydrate diet causes an increase in blood glucose or blood sugar which also directly inhibits immune cell function. The reason is that glucose and vitamin C are almost identical molecules. In fact, most mammals can produce their own vitamin C from glucose. This is why carnivores don't get scurvy.

Why does eating a high sugar meal suppress immune function?

Humans cannot make our own vitamin C. Vitamin C is thus an essential nutrient for humans. Because vitamin C and glucose are so similar they can actually bind to the same receptors on immune cells called phagocytes. If you have high blood sugar many of the receptors on your immune cells get bound to glucose and the vitamin C gets competitively inhibited from binding. This means that your immune cells cannot get the vitamin C they require and thus they cannot work properly. The solution is NOT to consume copious amounts of synthetic vitamin C (it is made from coal tar), it is to stop consuming so much carbohydrate and to reduce your allostatic load - move to a more genetically congruent environment – eat, move, and think in more genetically congruent ways.

A lot of bad things happen when humans consume a high carbohydrate, low fat diet. This type of diet is deadly for humans. In fact, during the past two decades that such a diet has been advocated by the "dietary experts", obesity rates have skyrocketed in both adults and children.

Just so you don't get misinformed, the exercise and energy expenditure patterns have not decreased during this time – we can't blame the increases in obesity on decreased activity levels.

There's not a hunter gatherer population anywhere in the world that eats a high carbohydrate, low fat diet. And there is not a hunter gatherer population anywhere in the world that has obesity or heart disease. In fact, research done on the Inuit, a population that subsisted on what was almost certainly the highest fat diet in human history, shows that these people had virtually no cardiovascular issues.[64] The Inuit, before they were convinced to eat a lower fat, higher carbohydrate diet, basically had a blubber breakfast, a 10:00 a.m. blubber snack, followed by a blubber lunch, a blubber afternoon snack, a blubber dinner, and a before-bed blubber snack.

You have to ask yourself where the food pyramid came from. Was it based on a whole bunch of research or was it based on grain and dairy lobbies? You need to ask yourself that. I'll answer these questions, with more evidence than you can imagine, in my next book. I have already answered these questions in my Innate Diet book but it is not really a lay-public friendly book to read so I am rewriting it in a more appropriate format. I'm busy!

"Two or more daily servings from each (of the four food groups) are now considered necessary for a balanced diet, but humans living before the development of agriculture and animal husbandry derived all their nutrients from the first two food groups (meats, fish and fruits and vegetables); they apparently consumed cereal grains rarely, if at all, and they had no dairy foods whatsoever."

Eaton & Konner 1985 Paleolithic Nutrition: a consideration of its nature and current implications. N.Eng. J. Med. 312, 283-289.

There are few things more harmful than sugar. There are few things more harmful than breakfast cereals, breads, and pasta. Cereals and pasta are sugar. I don't care if it is a complex carbohydrate or simple carbohydrate, it's irrelevant, the only relevant issue is whether or not it is genetically compatible. The human genome doesn't know what to do with grains and refined sugar and high fructose corn syrup because our ancestors just didn't consume it – our genes were formed long before we ever consumed refined sugars, cereals, breads and pastas. Our ancestors would have had to expend more energy collecting grains and cereals than they would have got from eating them. Why? Because cereal grains didn't grow in big

Who created the food pyramid? What research was this based upon?

fields like they do on agricultural farms.[65]

For the record our ancestors didn't have dairy either. They didn't chase a wildebeest around and suckle it or attach their baby to it. There was no dairy in the human diet when our genes were formed and dairy is NOT a genetically congruent food for humans.

Genetically, we have not changed for thousands of years, but our lifestyle has significantly changed. If you actually look at what's happened since the agricultural revolution 10,000 years ago, when we added grains to our diet, when we added all these Omega 6 fatty acids and took out all the Omega 3 fatty acids, the human brain has actually gotten smaller. The human brain has shrunk significantly since the agricultural revolution.

Did our healthy hunter-gatherer ancestors consume a low fat, high carbohydrate diet?

The United States, Canada, and all the Western nations are basically feed lots. We take a cow and make it obese and strip it of healthy omega 3 fatty acids and fill it full of unhealthy omega 6 fatty acids in six weeks by feeding it grain and not letting it exercise. We can make a cow obese in six weeks. These cows also get liver tumors. Up to 90 percent of those cows will get a liver tumor in those six weeks of eating grain.[66] Check out the feed lots. The rule on the feed lot is that if the cow is not ambulatory, meaning it can't walk, they can't slaughter it. So you know what they do? They lift them up on forklifts so they can stand, then they slaughter them. These cows are so sick in these feed lots because they're eating grain, and their bodies don't know how to digest grain because they're supposed to eat grass. Cows have a four chambered stomach designed to ferment grass not grain. When they eat grain they get so much gas they have to have tubes

"Brain size has actually declined since the Paleolithic: the current average, 1,350 cm^3, is about 11 percent less than estimates for early anatomically modern humans living before the development of agriculture."

Eaton et al. The return of n-3 fatty acids into the food supply. Land based animal food products and their health effects. 1998 World Rev. Nutr. Diet Vol 83, 12-23 stuffed into them to release the gas. This is what happens when you eat foods you are not genetically designed to eat. The same thing is happening to humans. We are fat, devoid of healthy omega 3 fatty acids, filled with unhealthy omega 6 fatty acids, and getting full of tumors. We are also gassy and wrought with digestive issues; humans get gassy when they eat grains, too (mostly men, apparently).

We essentially live in a feed lot; industrial society is a feedlot for humans. We eat grain and we sit around and get fat and get sick.

As for dairy, human beings are the only species on earth that would drink the milk from another mammal. Human beings are also the only species on earth that consumes milk past infancy. Human beings are also the only species on earth with osteoporosis. You keep getting told to drink more milk, drink more milk. Do you know there is not a single study anywhere that shows that drinking milk increases bone density? There is calcium in milk, but it doesn't increase bone density and it is NOT even naturally present because the cows don't eat grass anymore, they eat grain, which is not only devoid of calcium, it actually blocks the absorption of calcium.[67] THE CALCIUM CONTAINED IN MILK IS ADDED IN SUPPLEMENT FORM. Why would anyone drink milk for calcium when, even if calcium was the issue in osteoporosis which it is not, you could simply supplement with calcium for pennies a day in a calorie-free format. Milk is simply a calorie rich calcium supplement delivery system that does not increase bone density. Please go to www.wellnessandprevention.com and read my newsletter entitled 'The Myths of Calcium Supplementation and Dairy'.

Does consuming more protein automatically produce strong muscles? Does consuming more calcium automatically produce strong bones?

By the way, there are studies to show that if you eat more fruits and vegetables, and get calcium in the organic form you genetically require (and create more alkalinity in your body), you will increase bone density.[68] But the real question to be asked is, how are you going to get better bone density if you don't exercise? Do you think that you can sit around on your couch drinking protein shakes and get big muscles? Some of the recommendations of "experts" are just so unscientific and illogical that I just scratch my head and wonder how they have ever been incorporated into mainstream clinical practice. It actually frightens me sometimes. Osteoporosis is not an issue of a lack of calcium, it's an issue of a lack of laying calcium down in bone or keeping calcium in bone. You can't do either of these if you are sedentary or eat improperly. You need to consume genetically congruent foods and put your bones under tensile stress from exercise and gravity so that the physiological and biochemical pathways get epigenetically stimulated and have the proper materials to work with. Just the fractures from osteoporosis, not the drugs, none of the treatments for osteoporosis, but just dealing with the fractures costs $38 Million A DAY in the United States![69] All this in the midst of copious amounts of dairy consumption and calcium supplementation.

If they gave me $38 Million a day I could actually house, feed, and have personal trainers for everybody, and I would not only prevent osteoporosis I would save the system money as I did it. Sickness is the biggest industry on the planet, the figures are staggering.

Which is pathological, the environment full of stressors or the adaptive physiological responses necessary to survive these stressors?

As soon as you eat, move or think in a way that is not genetically congruent that's a stressor, a rock in your backpack and you are going to release stress hormones. The chronic release of these stress hormones, and the lifestyle and environmental stressors that lead to this release, cause a cascade of other physiological adaptations including insulin resistance, chronic inflammation, decreased sex hormone binding globulin, and down-regulated immune function. These are what I term the five physiological pillars of chronic illness. The most important thing I want you to understand is that all these physiological processes that drive us toward, and can result in, chronic illness, start with the exposure to chronic stressors, with rocks in our backpacks initiating the acute stress response. Further, I cannot emphasize enough that the physiological changes associated with the acute stress response are absolutely necessary for survival in a stressful environment. If you could not produce these changes you would not be able to survive acute stressors and you would die of acute illness long before you developed chronic illness.

HOWEVER, we are not designed to be under chronic stress. What was designed to be helpful in an acute fight or flight situation is now being stimulated for months and years. The physiological response is not pathological, it is intelligent and appropriate and necessary to survive in a stressful environment. It is the environment that is pathological, or perhaps, our decision to remain in it.

Staying on that iceberg is what's pathological. The body's

> "Prolonged deviations from "normal" values represent not an error but an attempted adaptation to circumstances. If the prolonged deviation from normal values represents a threat to health, in the allostatic view the better response is to "change the circumstances" instead of pharmacologically attempting to "clamp" the parameter to normal."
>
> Power, Michael. L. in Schulkin, Jay. (2004) Allostasis, Homeostasis, and the Costs of Physiological Adaptation. Cambridge University Press. Cambridge, U.K.

response to it is not pathological, and having the strategy of trying to change the body's intelligent response to stress by adding drugs that stop the body from being able to express a state of adaptive physiology is not only not working it is hindering our ability to prevent and recover from chronic illness.

Let's now summarize the physiological changes or adaptations associated with the alarm or adaptation response to stressors. This will allow us to better see how chronic stress becomes chronic illness. The physiological changes associated with exposure to chronic stressors can be summarized as follows:

What makes more sense, changing the pathological environment or using drugs to change our intelligent physiological adaptive response?

1. Increased cortisol
2. Increased catecholamines
3. Increased heart rate
4. Increased vasoconstriction
5. Increased blood pressure
6. Increased blood glucose levels
7. Increased blood lipid levels

8. Changed blood cholesterol profile (increased LDL cholesterol, decreased HDL cholesterol)

9. Increased blood clotting factors

10. Increased protein degradation of muscle and connective tissue

11. Insulin resistance (down regulated insulin receptors)

12. Increased feelings of stress, fear, anxiety and depression

13. Decreased short term memory, ability to concentrate, and learn new information

14. Decreased serotonin levels; increased noradrenaline levels

Are we genetically programmed to live under chronic stress or to pursue homeostatic environments?

15. Increased sensitivity of sensory systems including those for pain and other emotions

16. Down regulated cellular immunity

17. Decreased anabolic hormones like growth hormone and testosterone and luteinizing hormone etc

18. Bone loss, muscle fiber type changes, decreased R.E.M. sleep

What happens when we put ourselves in a chronic, pathological stressful environment is that we force our genes to adapt to this environment and to express chronic stress physiology. This is not a disease and it is not pathological – the chronically stressful environment is pathological NOT the body's response to it.

If we could not produce these changes we could not survive. But look what can result from being forced to adapt to this unnaturally stressful environment, this genetically incongruent environment for our species. These physiological changes were NEVER designed to be chronic. Chronically maintaining these adaptive states taxes our adaptability to the limit and places an allostatic load upon our

"Note that "adaptation" refers simply to the resetting of response sensitivity to a signal. Although it may turn out badly over time, the outcome is not caused by any low-level error or defect. Consequently it should not be considered as "inappropriate" or as "dysregulation".

"The allostasis model clearly identifies a paradox: people are dying, but their internal regulatory mechanisms are intact."

Sterling, Peter in Schulkin, Jay. (2004) Allostasis, Homeostasis, and the Costs of Physiological Adaptation. Cambridge University Press. Cambridge, U.K.

physiology; the inevitable result is physiological (cellular) fatigue and illness. The evidence that chronic stress and chronic allostatic load lead to chronic illness is overwhelming. Many studies have shown that allostatic load is a reliable predictor of both chronic illness and mortality.[70]

What are the major killers in industrial society? Heart disease, stroke, cancer, diabetes and the drugs prescribed to treat these "diseases of adaptation" or "lifestyle diseases". What are the major chronic problems? Depression, obesity, anxiety, fatigue, chronic pain, osteoporosis, fibromyalgia, lack of sleep, decreased sex drive, decreased fertility, indigestion, accelerated aging, ADHD, impotence and the side effects from the drugs prescribed to treat these problems. These are virtually all preventable. The best journals in the world are now stating that virtually all chronic diseases, including cancers, are preventable or lifestyle and immune function related. These are all lifestyle diseases caused by chronic exposure to stressors from living in genetically incongruent environments and choosing genetically incongruent lifestyle choices.

Look at the list of physiological changes like increased heart rate and blood pressure and vasoconstriction, increased fatty acids and glucose and clotting factors and chronic inflammation and ask yourself if this isn't heart disease and stroke waiting to happen.

What are the leading causes of death in industrial society? What are the leading causes of the leading causes of death in industrial society?

What about the increased stress hormone, decreased serotonin and decreased growth hormone levels which together produce depression, fatigue, and anxiety as well as memory, learning and attention deficits, as well as decreased sex drive and accelerated aging?

What about the insulin receptor resistance and increased blood glucose and blood lipid levels and fatigue and increased cravings and consumption of fatty and sugary foods leading to obesity and type II diabetes?

What about the chronically increased cortisol levels, suppressed immune function, decreased sex hormone binding globulin levels and cancer?

What about chronic increased cortisol levels, decreased growth hormone levels and osteoporosis?

What are "diseases of civilization" and "diseases of adaptation"?

Virtually every major health issue in society is addressed here. Dr. Hans Selye referred to these problems as "diseases of adaptation", Dr. Boyd Eaton refers to these illnesses as "diseases of civilization"; both are exactly right. I refer to these illnesses as "diseases of lifestyle" or "diseases of genetically incongruent environment". The fact is, regardless of the terminology, these illnesses are NOT genetic illnesses, they are NOT caused by inborn cellular pathology, and they ARE preventable.

The problem is that these facts are all but ignored within the Sickness & Treatment Paradigm and by the practitioners working within it. Let's look at what happens when drugs and surgery are seen as the solutions to lifestyle problems. Let's look at what happens when it is assumed that the genes are faulty or that the cell function is pathological. Let's look at what happens when the environment is ignored and success is measured by the ability to change adaptive physiology with drugs.

Let's take blood pressure as an example. Medicine takes a blood pressure reading and if it is higher than "normal" (what it would be in a relaxed environment) a toxic drug is prescribed. The goal of this toxic drug is to prevent the body from being able to raise blood pressure because they see high blood pressure as a disease or pathology rather than what it really is - an innately intelligent adaptation to a stressful environment.

"Second, the variables targeted for treatment are being driven to their particular levels by concerted signals from the brain in response to predicted needs. Consequently, if one signal is suppressed by a drug, the brain compensates by driving all the others harder. Thus, when blood pressure is treated by a diuretic to reduce volume, there are compensatory increases in heart rate and vasoconstriction. These can be treated in turn by beta-adrenergic antagonists, calcium channel antagonists, and so on. But adding more drugs to a complex system increases the frequency of iatrogenesis (illness caused by the treatments).

Sterling, Peter in Schulkin, Jay. (2004) Allostasis, Homeostasis, and the Costs of Physiological Adaptation. Cambridge University Press. Cambridge, U.K.

The drug results in lower blood pressure by shutting down normal adaptive physiological pathways (i.e. angiotensin converting enzyme inhibitors) and the medical doctor and the patient mistakenly feel like the treatment has resulted in increased health. Remember that the reason the innate genetic intelligence of the body appropriately elevated blood pressure was to deal with the increased energy demands of the stressful environment – it was an intelligent adaptation. When this is artificially over ridden with chemical toxins that prevent appropriate cell function, the innate genetic intelligence of the body via the central nervous system recognizes that blood pressure is inappropriately low given the demands from the stressful environment and responds by releasing more stress hormones in order to try and elevate the blood pressure to where it should be based on this environmental demand.

If we need increased blood pressure to deal with increased environmental demand under stress what happens when we take drugs that artificially lower blood pressure?

Blood pressure may artificially come down but the patient gets sicker from the diseases of adaptation that develop from the toxic and deficient lifestyle choices and the chronically increased stress hormone levels that have never been addressed and, worse, further aggravated. When another sign or symptom of their 'disease of adaptation' is discovered another drug is prescribed and the cycle of declining health and inclining medication continues.

Again, remember that the innate genetic intelligence of the body only increased blood pressure because of the increased energy demands associated with the increased stress or in order to adapt to an environmental stressor. The drugs inhibit this ability to adapt so the patient is left with even further decreased energy and often gets anxious or depressed. What does medicine do? Prescribe an antidepressant or anti-anxiety drug of course. Does the antidepressant cure the problem or even address the cause? NO. Now the person has artificially increased serotonin levels and becomes addicted to the anti-depressant that is documented to lose its effect and increase it's side effects with time.[71, 72] But what has happened to the normal physiological pathways responsible for regulating serotonin levels? They have been shut down or down regulated even further because of the feedback suppression loops. What happens to testicles if you take testosterone? They shrink because they are down regulated because of the feedback suppression loops.

Is it logical to assume someone is better or healthier simply because they have lowered blood pressure or cholesterol with a drug?

So now what happens if the patient stops taking these drugs? Blood pressure usually skyrockets if they get off the anti-hypertensive drugs because the body has released so much more stress hormone trying to increase blood pressure to where it should be. If they stop taking the anti-depressant they usually get drug withdrawal symptoms and even greater depression if they get off the serotonin reuptake inhibitors because their natural ability to produce serotonin has been shut off and they have had no interventions to stimulate the natural serotonin increasing and stress reducing pathways (i.e. the movement-pleasure pathways that exercise can help turn back on).

What about high cholesterol? Medicine has drugs for that too. Here again they can artificially lower cholesterol with a toxic drug that over rides normal physiology. Does this address the cause or make the patient healthier? No, it makes the patient have lower cholesterol levels which is all they measure so here again patient and doctor mistakenly feel like increased health has been accomplished. The joy for the patient is very often short lived as taking away the necessary increased cholesterol in a chronically stressful environment often leads to increased irritability and depression from the increased noradrenaline and cortisol that the body produces in an attempt to return the cholesterol levels to what is physiologically required to adapt to the stressful environment. What may be even more depressing is when the cholesterol medications cause muscle wasting and weakness and pain. Even more depressing is when the patient finds out that there is no evidence that taking these drugs prevents heart disease which is of course the reason they were prescribed in the first place. I'm getting depressed just writing about it.

Are patients given a test to determine if their regulatory systems are working improperly before they get prescribed a drug to over ride their regulatory systems?

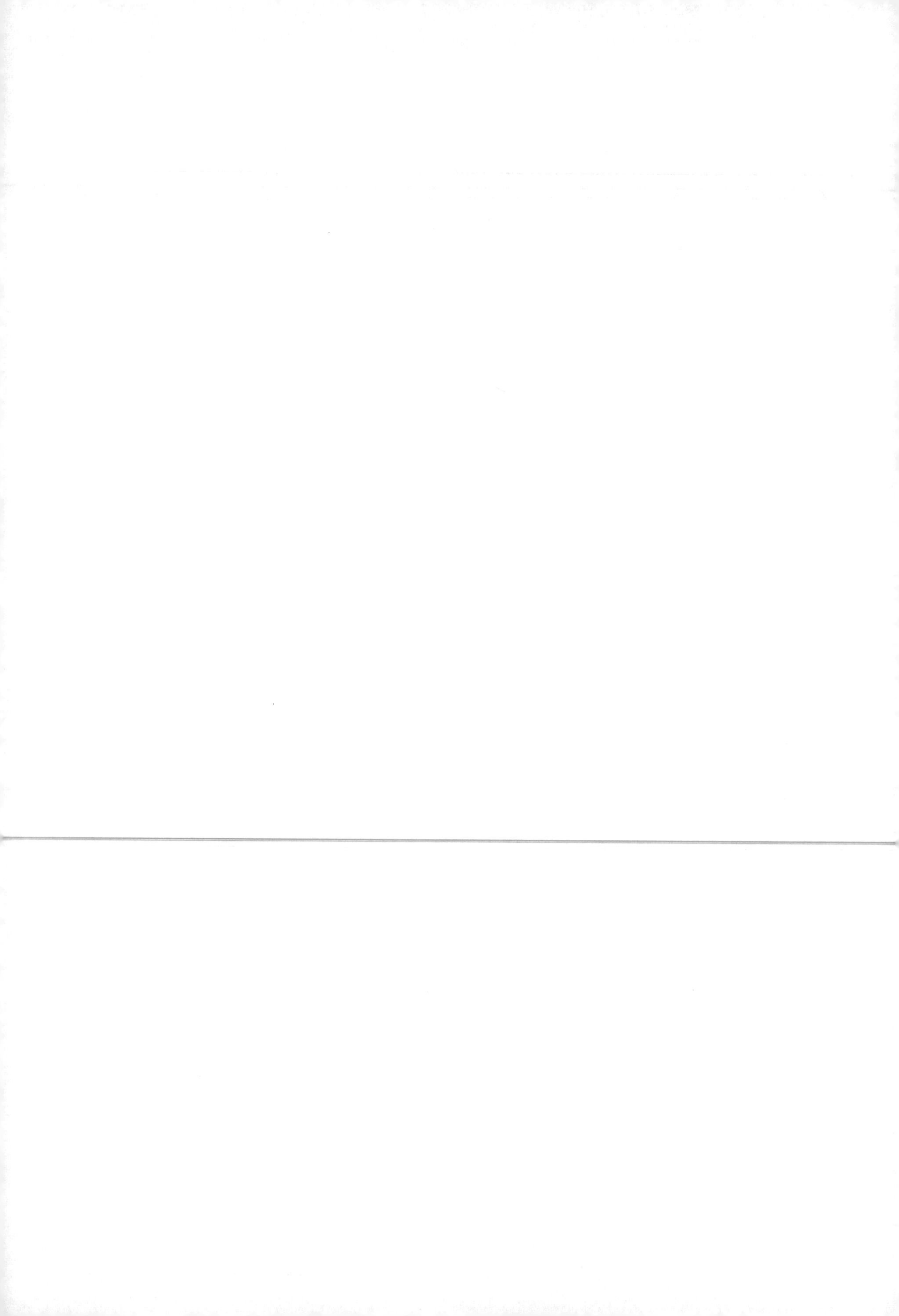

Chapter 7
How Do We Get and Stay Well: More Diagnosis, Drugs, and Surgery?

"Drugs never cure disease. They merely hush the voice of nature's protest, and pull down the danger signals she erects along the pathway of transgression. Any poison taken into the system has to be reckoned with later on even though it palliates present symptoms. Pain may disappear, but the patient is left in a worse condition, though unconscious of it at the time."

Daniel H. Kress, M.D.

At this point I feel you have enough information to accurately answer the first of the two most important questions regarding human health. That question is; why are humans so sick? I think you have seen enough evidence to conclude that humans are so sick with chronic illness because of our environment, because of our lifestyle choices. More specifically humans are so sick because we are living in ways that are genetically incompatible, we are eating, moving, thinking, and interacting in ways that are stressful and that place a chronic stress load or allostatic load on our physiology. We bio-accumulate the effects of our bad lifestyle choices and over time this catches up to us.

We are not sick because of bad genes or innately pathological cell function. We are not sick because of bad genes, bad cells, or bad luck. We are sick because of bad choices. We are sick because we have created, and choose to live in, pathologically stressful environments that force the chronic genetic expression of unsustainable adaptive physiology that inevitably leads to fatigue and early death.

We are now ready to answer the second of the two most important questions regarding human health; what is required to get and stay well? This is really the entire point of this book, to empower you to be able to answer this question. Remember, this book is not about assessing blame, this book is about taking responsibility. If you are going to develop the ability to take responsibility for your health you need to know what is required to get and stay well. The reason we spent so much time figuring out why we get chronic illness is because the answer to this question predetermines what solutions we will pursue to get and stay well. In fact, how we answer the first question predetermines whether or not we will even consider that it is possible to get and stay well.

The fact is that the prevailing Sickness & Treatment Paradigm is a belief system that assumes chronic illness is the result of bad genes, bad cells or bad luck and that the solution is more drugs and surgeries. That's just bad science and bad logic and it has produced bad results and is bankrupting nations, corporations and individuals.

If you wanted to sell drugs and surgeries what would you want people to believe, that chronic illness is caused by bad genes, bad cells, and bad luck or that chronic illness was caused by lifestyle choice?

If we believe we are sick due to genetic predetermination or to innately weak or pathological cells we will inevitably conclude that wellness and prevention are impossible and thus spend all our time, energy, and resources on diagnosis and treatment. As long as we believe that we develop a chronic illness because of bad genes, bad cells or bad luck, then we feel we have no power to influence our own health destiny. Once we believe this it is easy to believe that we have no responsibility in terms of our health and sickness. Once we have adopted this belief system we have, by definition, adopted a stance of helplessness and dependence. We simply live our lives waiting to see what will happen, waiting to see if we will be one of the few lucky ones or, when it comes to chronic illness, one of the many unlucky ones.

As it stands now, if we actually believe we have no responsibility or power to determine our own health destiny, we have virtually no chance of living our lives without chronic illness. What is more frightening is that these odds are getting worse every year. Can you think of a worse belief system in terms of trying to get people to change their lifestyle habits? Can you think of a better belief system if you are trying to get people to buy drugs and surgeries or herbs and tonics? This is not to say that you may never require a drug or surgical intervention, it just means that you have the ability to exponentially reduce that chance. What I want to get across to you, and what I will get across to you, is that only when you understand the truth about why you get sick will you be empowered to make intelligent choices about how to get and stay well.

Just in case you somehow still believe that drugs and surgeries, or perhaps some as of yet undiscovered new and improved drugs and surgeries, are the answer to what is required to get and stay well we should look at the available data regarding this conclusion and its application in society. Perhaps you think I am being alarmist. Perhaps you may still believe that it just is not possible that so many intelligent experts have gotten it wrong. Perhaps you still think that the solution is to reform the current system of diagnosing and treating chronic illness with drugs and surgery.

At this point I must ask you to ask yourself why you still think this. What evidence do you have that the current system is working to heal or prevent chronic illness? What evidence do you have to suggest the current system will ever work to heal or prevent chronic illness? Even if the current system could successfully treat chronic illness, which it most certainly cannot, how could we afford it? If more and more people get more and more chronic illness every year and require more and more treatments which cost more and more money how can this be sustained? It can't. Let me repeat what I said in the opening chapter. The ONLY solution to the current pandemic of chronic illness and the economic and social burdens it causes is fewer sick people (more healthy people).

Is there any available evidence that prescribing more drugs and performing more surgeries has increased health or decreased the incidence or prevalence of chronic illness? Where did you read that, may I have a copy?

The fact is that until we can create a population that has less illness per person we will never spend less per person, we will never have more productivity per person, we will never have more quality of life per person and we will always spend more per person.

Treating chronic illness NEVER saves money, treating chronic illness ALWAYS costs money. In fact, the earlier we intervene and start treatment the more it costs. Unless early intervention prevents the need for further intervention, early detection simply means that people start costing money earlier (or increasing profits earlier for those in the disease treatment business). Sick people become customers sooner. Think about it. What percentage of early detection and treatment results in a person getting cured and thus not requiring any more treatment? If prescribing more drugs and performing more surgeries got people better and saved money then what we would see is that if we spent more at the start we would begin to have to spend less. What we would see is that people who got treatment would get better and then no longer need treatment.

Let's look at the data, let's not guess, let's look at the actual published data and then come to a logical, scientific, evidence-based conclusion. Let's examine what has happened over the past 50 year period during which we have prescribed more drugs per person every year, performed more surgeries per person every year, spent more money on drugs and surgeries per person every year, and developed more chronic illness per person every year.

In the United States spending on prescription drugs alone increased by 55 times between 1960 and 2002. The health of the population steadily declined and illness rates steadily increased during the same period.

CRS Report for Congress.
Health Care Spending: Past trends and projections.
(Updated April 8, 2004)
Paulette C. Morgan

Does prescribing drugs reduce or increase the future need for prescribing drugs?

The data is clear. Prescribing more drugs, to more people, at earlier points in their lives, or to people in earlier states of disease, has NOT resulted in less sickness or less spending. The cost of treating sickness is increasing exponentially both on a per capita and per year basis.

Chronic illness is HUGELY expensive. How expensive. Let me break it down by disease to give you a better idea of the scope of this issue. Keep in mind, these figures, although posted or reported or published very recently, are often based on figures over a decade old. This means these are conservative figures. Spending on heart disease and stroke is reported to be $1.3 Billion; spending on cancer is reported to be $625 Million; spending on diabetes is reported to be $477 Million, spending on obesity is reported to be $402 Million, spending on digestive disorders is reported to be $337 Million, spending on just the fractures from osteoporosis is reported to be $38 Million.[73, 74, 75, 76, 77, 78, 79] Ladies and gentlemen these are PER DAY figures.

In 2002 spending on prescription drugs reached $3.5 billion PER DAY. This figure will be over $7 billion PER DAY by 2013.[80] This equates to $292 Million per hour and $4.9 Million per minute.

These figures are not only staggering they are, without any debate, unsustainable. There's no way we can keep this up. The most

> "Rising rates of chronic diseases pose a significant and growing problem in the United States. The incidence of chronic diseases has increased dramatically over the last three decades."
>
> Almanac of Chronic Disease, 2009 Partnership to Fight Chronic Disease

disturbing fact is that of all the money being spent, there is not a penny of it that is going to stop us from spending more in the future. There is nothing in the sickness treatment system that prevents chronic illness or spending on chronic illness. It is a positive feedback loop, it is self perpetuating. There's nothing in drugs and surgery that's going to prevent people from having heart disease, or cancer, or digestive disorders, or obesity, or diabetes, or arthritis. When you take those pills, you don't go away after two weeks and say, "Good, I'm done. I'm cured." You keep taking them. You're a customer for life, and not a longer, better life I might add. Remember, a million people died of heart disease in the U.S. last year. Were they the ones who forgot to take their pills? Did they get heart disease because they had a deficiency of pills? Does anyone have any chronic illness because they were born with a deficiency of drugs?

Is health care really free in countries where it is socialized?

By the way, these figures are consistent across virtually all industrial nations, including Canada, Australia, and Great Britain. In British Columbia, Canada, the healthiest spot in the world, we think, 42 percent of all government spending goes towards treating sickness. I love it when people from Canada or Australia, or Britain, or anywhere else with socialized medicine say, "Well, thank goodness we have free health care." Are you kidding me? Do you think the doctors work for free? Do the nurses work for free? Are the hospital buildings built for free? Are the drugs supplied to the pharmacies for free? Do the pharmacists work for free? Is all the equipment free? Then how have we come to believe we have free medical care? It's not free, it's just subversively funded by taxes. It comes out of the VERY high taxes we pay. Virtually half of every tax dollar collected goes to sickness care. They just convince people it is free so they don't investigate the real costs. Despite all these tax funds they still have to raise billions more in donations just to keep the system afloat and even this is not working - the system is sinking fast. As in all industrial nations with socialized sickness treatment, it is projected that by the year 2017 a full 70 percent of all tax revenue will be spent on sickness treatment. Over 80 percent of those monies will go to treating chronic illness. Today nearly 40 percent of all British Columbians have a chronic illness. According the provincial government, British Columbia alone spends $1.5 million on sickness PER HOUR.

Just for the record, during this period of exponential increase in chronic illness, prescription rates, and spending, the genes in these same populations have not changed. It is statistically and scientifically absurd to blame the increases in chronic illness rates on genes. If chronic illness rates are exponentially increasing and gene change is virtually a constant, how can we attribute increasing illness rates to genes? We can't. However, there have been exponential unhealthy changes in our lifestyle during this period of exponentially increasing chronic illness, prescription rates, and spending. I can tell you that, as our chronic illness rates have steadily increased, the changes away from what is matched to our genetic requirements in terms of environmental toxins and how we eat, move, think, and interact have matched this increase.

Is providing more access to more drugs and surgeries to more people a logical approach to health care reform?

As I quoted in an earlier chapter from the World Health Organization, the current modern industrial diet was unknown to our ancestors just a few generations ago and is MUCH less healthy and MUCH less matched to our genetic requirements for expressing health and preventing chronic illness.

Our energy expenditure (exercise) levels have decreased by 65 percent since World War II and a full 24 percent of Americans now have no daily exercise. [81]

Our emotional stress levels have skyrocketed and our sense of community and belonging has plummeted. The increases in chronic illness are directly attributable to the documented unhealthy changes in our lifestyle, particularly in the areas of pollutants, nutrition, exercise, and emotional stress. It is scientifically and statistically absurd not to attribute the increases in chronic illness to unhealthy lifestyle changes.

As horrifying as these data are regarding the expenditures on chronic illness the data that show that this is NOT working is even

Before we debate about how to pay for more drugs and surgery should we not first debate about whether or not they are working?

"Aggregate state spending on Medicaid increased from $89 billion in 2000 to $151 billion in 2007, leaving less money for education and infrastructure needs. However, higher-intensity care generally does not improve survival, and complications of medical care accounted for 1.1 million hospitalizations in 2006 – costing nearly $42 billion."

Kilo & Larson. 2009. Exploring the harmful effects of health care. JAMA Vol 302: No 1.

more disturbing. The elephant in the room during all the discussions on healthcare reform and healthcare spending reform, and health insurance reform, is that what we are paying trillions of dollars for is NOT working. I'm quite sure that President Obama has wonderful intentions regarding the health of the citizens he governs. I'm sure he actually believes that his Obama Care plan that gives 30 million more people access to drugs and surgeries will result in better health for his beloved citizenry. Let's stop the misleading debate about who should pay for this or if it is possible to pay for this. None of this is relevant. Let's ask if this will result in better health and less chronic illness. This is the relevant question.

What I don't understand is how someone as intelligent as President Obama, or all the other intelligent people involved in the healthcare debates, could have missed asking the most important question regarding healthcare reform. That is, "do more drugs and surgeries, more medical interventions (medical interventions are drugs and surgeries), result in better health and less sickness and thus reduce the need for future expenditures." Seems like a pretty obvious question to me. However, if you view this issue from within the Sickness & Treatment Paradigm, or are being advised by those who do, you operate under the a priori assumption that more drugs and surgeries will of course increase health and decrease chronic illness. You may also simply believe that, although they don't increase health or decrease chronic illness, drugs and surgeries are the only option to palliate the people who inevitably develop chronic illness due to bad genes, bad cells, or bad luck.

Let's figure out if more drugs and surgeries have ever resulted, or can sanely be expected to ever result, in increased health and decreased chronic illness and thus reduce future need for expenditure on chronic illness treatments.

Now, if I were in charge, BEFORE I offered more drugs and surgeries to 30 million more people, or committed to continue to offer these to a hundred million people, the question I would ask would be this. "Is there any data to show that this approach works? Has this approach worked for the hundreds of millions of people with chronic illness that have had access to drugs and surgeries over the past fifty years?"

Once again let's look at the data. If spending money on drugs and surgery made a population healthier then what we would see is that those populations with the most access to drugs and surgeries, those populations with the most use of and thus expenditures on drugs and surgeries, would have the best health. The fact is that the countries that spend the most money PER CAPITA on drugs consistently have the lowest health ratings. As Rippe et al. (2009) point out, "Every other industrialized economy that expends less money (on drugs and surgery) than the U.S. also achieve better health outcomes."[82]

Why have detailed cost-benefit analyses of drug and surgical care not been performed? How is it possible, without solid evidence for effectiveness, that they demand and receive so much funding?

In a recently published article in the Journal of the *American Medical Association* titled 'Exploring the harmful effects of health care' authors Kilo and Larson question the assumption that drugs and surgeries have a positive effect on health outcomes. In fact, they clearly point out that "the aggregate effect on health may be smaller than generally assumed."[83] Most importantly they point out that, because of this assumed benefit, scientific cost-benefit analyses are not being conducted. After looking

"Increases in the prevalence and treatment intensity of chronic disease are responsible for about two-thirds of the increase in health care costs over the past two decades."

Source: Thorpe K. The Rise In Health Care Spending And What To Do About It. Health Affairs. 2005;6:1436-1445. Also, Thorpe K, Florence CS, Joski P. Which Medical Conditions Account For The Rise In Health Care Spending?

at the data they point out that "the benefits that U.S. healthcare currently delivers may not outweigh the aggregate health harm it imparts." "Medicare spending shows wide per-capita variability across the United States, with patients receiving 60 percent more care in high-cost than in low-cost cities. Paradoxically, patients in higher-cost cities are more likely to die of colon cancer, myocardial infarction, and hip fracture."[84]

In a two part series published in the *Annals of Internal Medicine* Dr. Elliot Fisher, professor of medicine at Dartmouth University, comes to the same conclusions and points out that the assumption that more drugs and surgeries equate to better health outcomes is indeed false. He summarizes the findings of his scientific study regarding the costs and benefits of the current medical approach in a Dec 1, New York Times article as follows: "Our study suggests that perhaps a third of medical spending is now devoted to services that don't appear to improve health or quality of care – and may make things worse."

Who is responsible for the adverse effects and ineffectiveness of treatments? Who is liable?

To put that statement in perspective that means than on an annual basis as much as 1.4 trillion dollars is spent with no benefit. Thus, the cost of these ineffective treatments equates to $4 Billion PER DAY, $165 Millon PER HOUR, or $2.7 Million per Minute.

Those figures do not include any of the expenditure on addressing the harm or on the human costs of ineffective and/or harmful treatments. I have deliberately stayed away from the data on medical harm because I don't want this book to be about blame. Medicine is not responsible for chronic illness. However, all practitioners are responsible for the advice they give, the treatments they offer, and the fees they charge. If you are interested in learning more about the adverse effects of prescription drugs, the millions of hospitalizations this causes, the hundreds of thousands of deaths, and the billions of dollars it all costs you can read about this important and alarming issue elsewhere. This book is written so you can take responsibility for the advice you take, the solutions you choose, the fees you pay, and who you pay those fees to.

In 2020, if the current trends continue, the vast majority of our kids will be obese by the time they are 13 years old; not 50

> "The diagnosis of childhood chronic diseases has almost quadrupled over the past four decades."
>
> Perrin J, Bloom S, Gortmaker S. The Increase of Childhood Chronic Conditions in the United States. Journal of the American Medical Association. June 27, 2007.

percent of our kids as is the case now, but a vast majority will be obese. They will have Type 2 diabetes. They will be developing heart disease and cancer. More and more will have asthma and allergies and atopic disorders. More and more will have attention and behavior problems. They will watch television or play video games most of their waking hours. As hard as it is to believe or admit, these are the trends that the data clearly indicate. These statistics are NOT unique to the United States or North America. These statistics are highly representative of the entire human population living in industrialized nations.

If chronic illness was caused by genes and by aging, would reducing the rate of incidence, expenditure, or death be possible?

How can anyone look at this data and conclude that the solution is more drugs and surgery? Once we see the data there can be no debate about the facts that expenditures on chronic illness are increasing exponentially and that this has not decreased, and will not ever decrease, the incidence of chronic illness. However, if you believe that humans are genetically predetermined to get sick or that getting older causes heart disease, cancer, obesity, diabetes, digestive disorders, depression and dementia, then you would simply conclude that this increase in expenditure is inevitable. You would conclude that as our population increases, and as our population ages, we will inevitably just require more money for chronic illness. This is exactly what those within the Sickness & Treatment Paradigm do believe and exactly the message they disseminate to patients, politicians and policy makers.

I fully agree that IF chronic illness is caused by genes and aging then we are doomed to spend more money every year until, as the experts report in the literature, by the year 2043 we will be forced to spend every cent of every tax dollar treating chronic illness.[85] Yes, you read that correctly, by 2043, if trends continue, there will be no money for education, for roads or any other infrastructure, for pensions, for parks, or for any other government service. Still, as bleak as this sounds, IF the Sickness & Treatment Paradigm is accurate, there is nothing we can do about this - we are on a predetermined and unalterable path. We may be able to do some healthcare reform to make the system a few percentage points more efficient but the result will be the same.

However, if you look at this issue through the Wellness & Prevention Paradigm you begin to ask some self evidently important questions. What about the fact that expenditure rates are increasing at exponentially higher rates than the population is increasing or aging? Remember, the percentage of the population aged 65 or older has not increased at all between 1990 and 2010 so aging has nothing to do with the per capita increases in chronic illness rates or expenditures. What about the fact that per capita expenditures are increasing exponentially? What about the fact that per capita prescription rates are increasing exponentially? What about the fact that pharmaceutical company profits are rising exponentially? What about the fact that adverse effects, hospitalizations, and deaths from correctly prescribed prescription drugs are rising exponentially? What about the fact that chronic illness rates are rising exponentially faster than genes can change or the population is aging? What about the fact chronic illness is rising exponentially in our children and middle aged populations?

Should health care reform be about reforming how we pay for the ever increasing demand for drugs and surgery or should health care reform be about reforming what interventions are offered and paid for?

Is it not possible, in fact highly probable, in fact indisputable, that the hypotheses regarding why we are sick put forward by those within the Sickness & Treatment Paradigm have been disproven yet not discarded and that this is the underlying cause of the increasing expenditures in the midst of increasing chronic illness? Is it not possible, in fact highly probable, in fact indisputable, that treating the effects of lifestyle caused illnesses with drugs and surgeries instead of addressing the lifestyle causal factors is the real issue that nobody seems to want to address?

Is it not time to speak about reforming what kind of care is offered rather than trying to reform how to continue to offer drugs and surgeries? YES!

Recently I had a very interesting experience. I was invited to Missouri to speak to a large insurance group. I was asked to come and present to the group in the hopes that they would become informed about the importance of lifestyle with respect to wellness and prevention and quality of life and thus become inspired to make healthy changes. I am getting more and more of these requests from corporations.

The fact is that abundant sickness and scarce health is the biggest issue facing employers, employees, and those that provide health insurance.

None of this was out of the ordinary. What was extraordinary from my perspective was the fact that none of the data I shared was shocking to any of the people in the insurance business. Yes it shocked some of the employees but the people in the insurance industry, the people who have more data than anyone in the world on chronic illness and the costs associated with it, were not only familiar with my data on illness and expenditure rates but had been so for decades. Let me explain.

If two people have the same "normal" reading for blood pressure or cholesterol but one is taking blood pressure or cholesterol drugs are they equally healthy?

One of the things I often point out to practitioners is the fact that when an insurance company determines what the premiums will be for health insurance they do not do so by random chance. NOTHING an insurance company does is determined by random chance. Insurance companies have actuaries that spend their careers looking at data trends. This is how they figure out what to charge for premiums. They need to know what risk someone is for making a claim. They need to know what the odds are that someone will make a claim over the next 5, 10, 15, 20 years. They also need to figure out exactly how much this claim is going to cost them. Without these figures they cannot determine what to charge for premiums in order to make sure they can cover all the claims and still make a profit.

This is not unethical, it is intelligent. Imagine if you were a house insurance company and you were going to offer fire insurance. How would you know what to charge? You would have to figure out what percentage of houses were going to have a fire and what this would cost you. From here you could figure out what premium rates you would need to charge based upon any given number of houses or clients you insured. It's all about the odds. Imagine if 80 percent of the houses you covered had a fire! You would go bankrupt UNLESS you increased the premiums high enough to cover these costs. Imagine how high the premiums would be.

Welcome to the health insurance business. The fact is that 80 percent of the working population now has a diagnosed chronic illness and 55 percent have more than one diagnosed chronic illness – I shared this data with you in an earlier chapter. Do you now understand why premiums are getting so high? Yes there is waste and yes we can make things more efficient but I don't care how efficient you make the system – if 80 percent of the people you cover make claims it is not sustainable.

It gets more interesting. Health insurance companies can figure out, almost to the decimal point, the chances of someone making a claim. How do they do this? They do it by calculating risk using risk factors such as body mass index, cholesterol level, blood pressure, whether someone smokes or if they already have a diagnosed illness etc. In fact, what they really do is calculate your stress load or your allostatic load, the number of rocks in your backpack, at the time you want to get coverage. From this they can predict whether or not and how often you will make a claim and cost them money.

If two people have the same "normal" reading for blood pressure or cholesterol but one is taking blood pressure or cholesterol drugs which one would pay higher health insurance claims? Why?

Here is the real kicker. Do you know that if two people have the exact same profile on the risk factors that they do not necessarily get charged the same premium? Did you know that if one person is on medication, if one person is receiving the gold standard medical intervention, and the other one is not, that the person receiving the medical care is a HIGHER risk in terms of illness and expenditure? Stop and think about that for a moment. If both people have "normal" blood pressure and cholesterol measurements but one person is using prescription drugs to attain those levels that person is statistically more likely to get sick, to get chronic illness, and to make more claims for future drugs and surgery. In other words, the fact that they are receiving drugs and surgery to treat the risk factors or to treat chronic illness does not make them healthy and the insurance companies have more data than you could ever sift through to prove this.

BINGO. This is where I come in, this is where the Wellness & Prevention Paradigm comes in. What the insurance companies and the employers have realized is that the system is unsustainable because the interventions don't make people well or prevent future illness – they just continue to cost more and more as people get sicker and sicker. There is no return on investment in terms of health, finances, employee or client satisfaction, or productivity. In the past when very few people were making claims this was not such a pressing issue.

If only 10 percent of the people you cover make claims, even if the interventions you pay for don't work, they are still affordable. However, as chronic illness rates have risen, this has become unsustainable and addressing the issue has become unavoidable.

Guess what these people have come to realize? They have come to realize that more drugs and surgeries are not the answer. They have come to realize that the only way to make things viable is to have fewer people making claims. They have come to realize that, regardless of what they spend on drugs and surgery, this has never and will never result in fewer people making claims because it does not result in fewer people being sick.

Having more healthy people making fewer claims is the ONLY viable solution and that's why I got the call. They needed someone with clinical expertise in Wellness & Prevention, they needed someone with expertise in how to get and stay well. Who doesn't? Really, who doesn't need such an expert?

What is the only way to reduce healthcare claims and costs - more treatment or less sickness?

I was also surprised, pleasantly surprised I might add, to find out that the wellness officer for this insurance group was a lifestyle-centric chiropractor. I guess it made sense really, what would be the point of having a drugs and surgery expert in charge of wellness and prevention? Anyway the evidence I shared about the ability of lifestyle change to prevent chronic illness, to heal from chronic illness, and to improve productivity and quality of life for the employees was a shock to everyone in the room (except the lifestyle centric chiropractor of course – this is why he advocated to have me come). Although the insurance experts were fully aware of the costs of drugs and surgery and the fact that they were not the solution they had never been exposed to the data I had regarding just how effective healthy lifestyle change can be. Further, the employees, the people the insurance company was providing coverage for, and charging premiums to, also realized how vital taking responsibility for their health was. At the end of the day it is meaningless to have unlimited coverage for treatment and remain ill and have a poor quality of life. EVERYONE wants a better, longer life and EVERYONE in that room, and I hope everyone reading this book, and soon EVERYONE on the planet, realizes that healthy lifestyle change is the only viable solution.

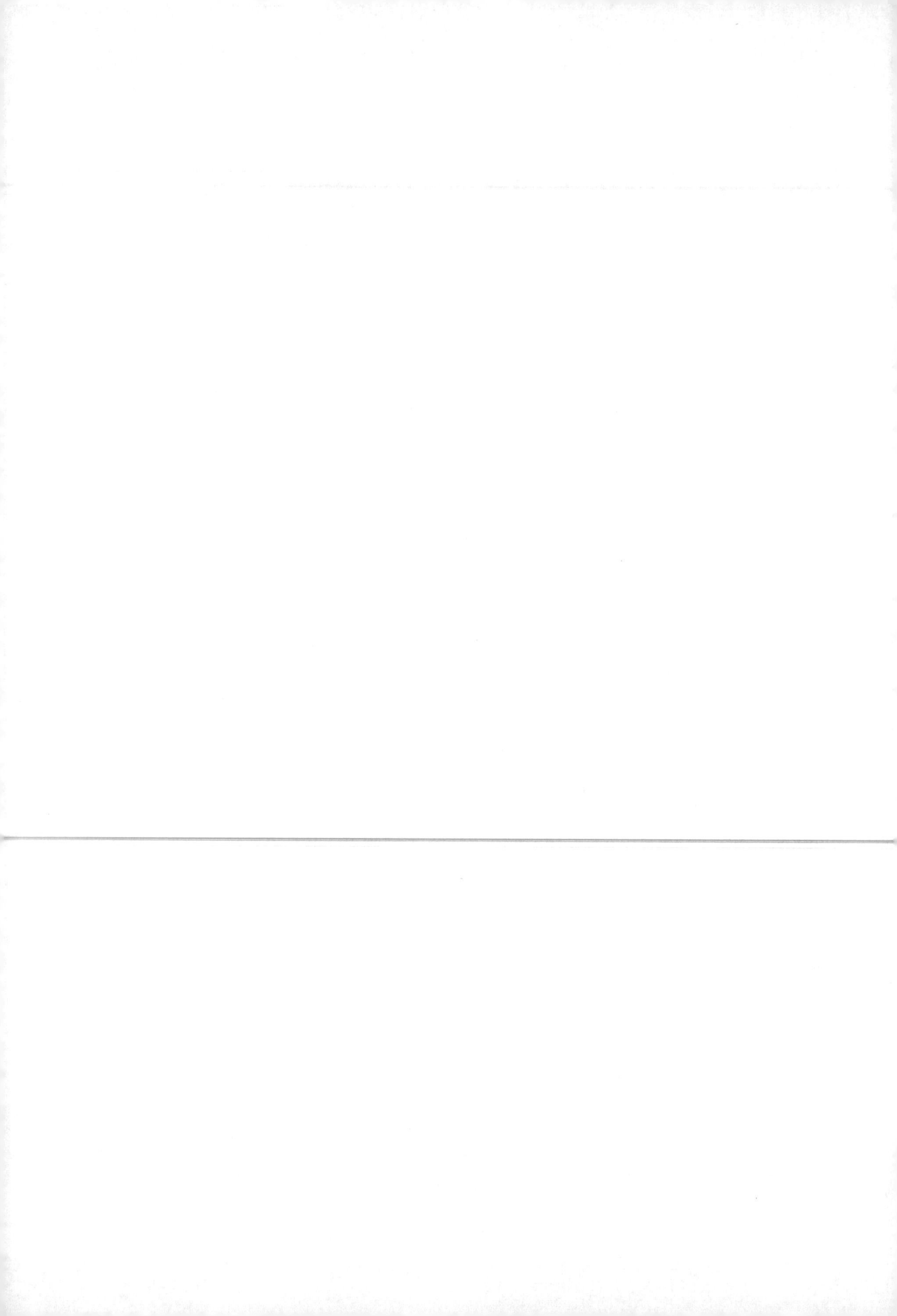

Chapter 8
How To Get and Stay Well: Evidence-Based Lifestyle Intervention

"The doctor of the future will give no medicine, but will interest patients in the care of the human frame, in diet, and the cause and prevention of disease."

Thomas Edison

"Nature's biological imperative is simple: No intelligence or ability will unfold until, or unless, it is given the appropriate model environment."

Eric Jensen (1995)
Brain-Based Learning

It is now time for the most important section of the book, the solution! It is time to substantiate that lifestyle is the only evidence-based, cost-effective solution for wellness and prevention. I want to leave you with certainty about the importance of your lifestyle choices and the amount of power and control you have regarding your own health destiny. I truly believe that, when you learn how significant your choices regarding how you eat, move, think, and interact are in terms of your health and your ability to prevent illness, that this information will create significant enough change in your belief systems to create meaningful change in your behaviors.

Let's spend some time reviewing the literature. Most of you will have some understanding regarding how certain lifestyle patterns can increase your chances of developing chronic illness but few of you will be aware of how important lifestyle choice is with regard to not only preventing illness, but to expressing your potential for health and vitality and for experiencing a better, longer, life. The research is unequivocal, lifestyle choices are the single greatest determinant of both quantity and quality of life.

Adopting a healthy lifestyle, a genetically congruent lifestyle, is the only viable solution for wellness and prevention. It is also the most evidence-based healing solution for those already suffering with chronic illness, and it SAVES LIVES, SAVES MONEY, and can SAVE HEALTHCARE.

In a recent article, I think the breakthrough landmark paper regarding the paradigm shift from Sickness & Treatment to Wellness & Prevention, Hyman et al. (2009) emphatically state that lifestyle needs to become the foundation of all healthcare.[86] They point out that for just the five most expensive chronic illnesses, heart disease, diabetes, metabolic syndrome, prostate cancer, and breast cancer, that addressing the lifestyle causes of these illnesses rather than treating them with drugs and surgery could not only save millions of lives but trillions of dollars.

Hyman et al. conclude that 1.9 TRILLION dollars could be saved on the treatment of these illnesses alone because adopting a healthy lifestyle PREVENTS illness and gets sick people well.[87]

Just imagine the human suffering that can be prevented; the money is insignificant when you compare it to the suffering.

Based on the literature, what is the most evidence-based intervention for preventing and healing from chronic illness?

More importantly is that these authors echo exactly what I pointed out years ago in my series of Innate Diet, Physical Fitness, and State of Mind books. They explain why drugs aimed at treating the effects of lifestyle-caused illnesses do not work. They articulate what I have been teaching for years, that chronic illness is lifestyle illness and simply giving drugs to alter the risk factors like blood pressure or cholesterol does not work. They make it clear to the reader that "lifestyle and environment influence the fundamental biological mechanisms leading to disease: changes in gene expression, which modulate inflammation, oxidative stress, and metabolic dysfunction."[88] Now I would not call it metabolic dysfunction, I would call it fatigue from chronic adaptation to a pathological environment but I can't tell you how wonderful it is to see this paradigm shift occurring.

"Lifestyle and environment influence the fundamental biological mechanisms leading to disease: changes in gene expression, which modulate inflammation, oxidative stress, and metabolic dysfunction."[89]

They actually state in this paper exactly what I have stated so many times in my books, from stage, on radio, on video, and taught to thousands of chiropractors in my post-graduate wellness lifestyle certification program. The changes in physiology associated with chronic illness are not genetic or pathological, they are epigenetic, they are the effects of environmental stressors. Remember what I taught you earlier, "your health or cell function is the genetic expression of your environment." Hyman et al. state,"The distinction between risk factors and causes is an important one. High blood pressure, dyslipidemia (high cholesterol), and elevated C-reactive protein (chronic inflammation) or glucose (insulin resistance) are not in and of themselves the real causes of chronic disease but simply surrogate markers that are the effects of environmental toxins, what we eat, how much we exercise, and how we respond to stress."[90] I nearly fell off my airplane seat when I read this, I wasn't sure whether to be happy that this paradigm shift is occurring or upset that I wasn't given any acknowledgement for having written the same thing years earlier! I know it's not about me.

> "There is strong evidence that this approach works and saves money. Unfortunately, insurance doesn't usually pay for it. No one profits from lifestyle so it is not part of medical education and practice."
>
> Hyman et al. Lifestyle Medicine: Treating the Causes of Disease. Alternative Therapies in Health and Medicine Nov/Dec 2010

Why isn't lifestyle part of medical education or part of the medical scope of practice?

These authors make some of the strongest statements I have ever seen get published in the peer-reviewed clinical literature. Even though this paper was published in an "alternative therapies" journal it is still an indication of how a paradigm shift is occurring. Hard to believe that lifestyle is considered "alternative". These authors not only espouse the importance of lifestyle, "It should be the foundation of our healthcare system", they also discuss the reasons it is not. "There is strong evidence that this approach works and saves money. Unfortunately, insurance doesn't usually pay for it. No one profits from lifestyle so it is not part of medical education and practice."[91]

This is exactly why we should not be relying on medical practitioners for expertise, advice, or interventions for wellness and prevention; it is simply outside their scope of education and practice.

By the way, this is true of most practitioners. Virtually all health care practitioners, in every field, are educated within the Sickness & Treatment Paradigm. This is precisely why I developed the post-graduate wellness lifestyle program – there was no other such program for chiropractors or any other health practitioners available. Where was the lack of trained wellness lifestyle practitioners leaving patients? With drugs and surgery of course.

One last series of quotes from this paper, I just feel it is such a landmark publication and as a scientist I cannot shake the engrained training that quoting the literature is more powerful than simply making the statement myself. I really enjoyed the way these authors directly compared and contrasted the current Sickness & Treatment approach to the proposed Wellness & Prevention approach. In fact I very rarely see anyone other than myself doing this so blatantly, most are constrained by fear of reprisal. Here is what they published.

If there are no wellness and prevention lifestyle practitioners where does this leave us, or, more importantly, what alternatives does this leave us with?

"Presently, according to the American Heart Association, 1.3 million coronary angioplasty and 448,000 coronary bypass operations are performed annually at a cost of more than $100 billion. Despite these costs, many studies, including one last month in the New England Journal of Medicine, reveal that angioplasties and stents do not prolong life or even prevent heart attacks in stable patients (ie 95 percent of those who receive them). Coronary bypass surgery prolongs life in less than 2 percent to 3 percent of patients who receive it."[92]

"In the ACCORD study of more than 10,000 diabetics, aggressive blood sugar lowering actually caused deaths. High blood sugar is a side effect of poor lifestyle choices. The treatment isn't insulin to lower blood glucose, but healthy dietary choices, exercise, stress management, and not smoking." [93]

"In contrast, the INTERHEART study, published in The Lancet in 2004, followed 30,000 people and found that changing lifestyle could prevent at least 90 percent of all heart disease."[94] No drug or surgery has ever, or will ever, be able to come close to this benefit. Yet drugs and surgery still dominate medical education and clinical intervention. How do these interventions get approved and incorporated as standard procedures if they don't work? The answer, as always, is profit and paradigm. The truth is that these procedures do work with regard to the outcome measures they test (change in blood flow after a stent or blood sugar levels for example). The problem is they don't work in terms of increasing health or prolonging life and they also often do great harm. Remember the plant analogy? It's all about what questions we ask and how we define better isn't it? It's all about paradigm. Perhaps the Center for Disease Control says it best, "Despite this evidence, our health care system has primarily focused on discovering treatments and cures for disease—not on preventing disease. In short, our health care system is not designed to prevent chronic illnesses."[95]

If we are told a drug "works" does this mean it works to increase health or to prevent disease or does it mean it "works" to change the single physiological variable they chose to target?

Let me now summarize some of the other literature providing evidence for the importance and effectiveness of lifestyle intervention. One of the most powerful clinical studies I have ever seen published is from Dr. Ornish. Dr. Ornish took patients with diagnosed prostate cancer and put them through a three month lifestyle program that included changes in diet, a 30 minute daily walk, and an hour of stress reduction in the form of breathing, meditation and imagery.[96] The results? The patients lost weight, reduced blood pressure and saw many other health improvements. What was most surprising to many was that they found changes in genetic expression (epigenetics) in about 500 genes.

The gene expression patterns of these men with prostate cancer actually shifted away from the pattern seen in cancer and toward a pattern reflecting wellness and prevention. More evidence that gene expression and illness are the result of lifestyle.[97]

One of my favorite review articles was written by Roberts and Barnard and published in 2005 in the Journal of Applied Physiology. I won't go into great detail but I will include a quote that I use often when I am lecturing, I think it is very powerful, especially when you consider it is published in perhaps the most respected journal in the world regarding human function.

"Currently, modern chronic diseases, including cardiovascular diseases, Type 2 diabetes, metabolic syndrome, and cancer are the leading killers in Westernized society and are increasing rampantly in developing nations. In fact, obesity, diabetes, and hypertension are now even commonplace in children. Clearly, however, there is a solution to this epidemic of metabolic disease that is inundating today's societies worldwide: exercise and diet."[98]

Perhaps the most thorough review of the benefits of lifestyle, at least in terms of exercising or moving well, was written by Booth et al. in 2002. This paper was also published in the Journal of Applied Physiology. Not only do these authors state that exercise is a genetic requirement for humans to express health and prevent illness, they also make it clear that the chronic illness physiology associated with sedentary living is not the result of bad genes or pathological cell function but rather due to living a genetically incongruent lifestyle.[99] Following is a summary of the benefits of incorporating exercise into our lifestyle which they cite in their paper. As you read about these amazing benefits keep this in mind. Most of these benefits are based on a 30 minute brisk walk and the research shows that the benefits of exercise are dose responsive meaning that the more you do the better. What this really means is that although 30 minutes of walking provides amazing benefit, it does not represent sufficiency with regard to the human genetic blueprint.

Documented Benefits of Walking:

What is meant by the statement that the benefits of exercise are dose responsive?

- Prevent up to 91 percent of cases of obesity and Type 2 diabetes
- Prevent up to 50 percent of all cases of heart disease
- Reduce risk of stroke by 25-30 percent
- Prevent up to 50 percent of all stroke deaths
- Reduce congestive heart disease deaths by 63 percent
- Reduce hospital readmission for heart failure patients by 70 percent
- Normalize blood pressure and reduce risk of developing high blood pressure
- Restore or maintain heart and blood vessel health
- Restore and maintain normal cholesterol triglyceride levels
- Reduce risk of breast cancer by up to 60 percent

- Reduce pancreatic cancer in overweight people by 50 percent
- Reduce lung cancer, even in smokers, by 72 percent
- Reduce melanoma, that's right, skin cancer apparently from the sun, by over 72 percent
- Prevent up to 50 percent of colon cancer
- Reduce risk of developing, and improve outcomes of those with, rheumatoid arthritis and osteoarthritis
- Prevent osteoporosis and increase new bone formation
- Increase strength, flexibility and balance
- Decrease gallbladder removal by 20 percent and decrease gallstones
- Improve digestion and decrease indigestion
- Improve bowel function and elimination
- Increase immune system function
- Increase macrophage (anti-tumor) activity and antioxidant levels
- Decrease all causes of mortality by 67 percent in the general population
- Decrease all-cause mortality by 50 percent in the 61 to 81 year-old age group
- Prevent up to 47 percent of cognitive impairment, prevent up to 62 percent of Alzheimer's and 52 percent of dementia
- Improve physical function in older adults
- Decrease chance of ever being in a nursing home
- Decrease rate of aging

How can one intervention like exercise be an evidence-based treatment for such a wide array of illnesses? Does exercise treat the illness or improve the health and function of the person with the illness?

- Enhance learning by 12 times
- Increase dopamine and serotonin levels
- Decrease depression by 20 percent, including relapses
- Increased growth and healing hormones
- Decrease stress and body breakdown hormones
- Decrease body fat, obesity, and weight gain

What drug or surgery could ever compete with these documented benefits? How much does a walk cost? How many lives could walking save? How much money could walking save? How can walking not be MANDATORY in our schools and workplaces? I hope you are amazed, I hope you are inspired to walk your way to a better, longer, life. Please don't forget to take your family, friends, and coworkers. So you know, I wrote this entire book (other than when I was in an airplane traveling to lecture) on a treadmill work station not sitting at a desk!

How can exercise prevent so many different types of conditions? Is exercise a panacea?

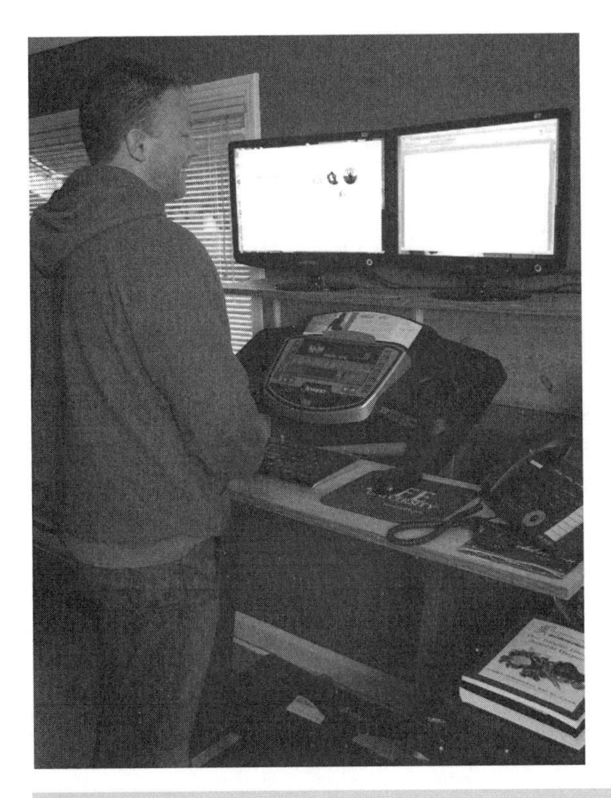

There are literally thousands of published peer-reviewed studies documenting the health and preventive benefits of consuming fruits and vegetables. Increasing fruit and vegetable intake increases sufficiency of genetically required nutrients and thus increases overall health and function. This is why eating fruits and vegetables is linked to prevention of virtually every illness and risk factor from cancer, to heart disease and stroke, to inflammation, to cholesterol levels, to blood pressure, to cognition, to digestion etc.

The Journal of Cancer, Epidemiology, Biomarkers & Prevention reported in 1996 that men who eat fresh fruit every day had a 70 percent less chance of dying from cancer of the digestive tract than those who ate almost no fruit.[100]

What is the only way for corporations to improve the health and productivity of employees and reduce the costs associated with chronic illness?

There is also ample evidence that lifestyle intervention works in the real world, that it is a practical approach. The Center for Disease Control reports "We have indisputable evidence of the power of prevention. Researchers and practitioners at national, state, and local levels have designed, tested, and implemented effective programs and policies for chronic disease prevention and control, many at very little cost."[101]

The *Partnership to Fight Chronic Disease 2009 Almanac of Chronic Disease* reports that "The Trust for America's Health estimates that an investment of $10 per person per year in community-based programs tackling physical inactivity, poor nutrition, and smoking could yield more than $16 billion in medical cost savings annually within 5 years. This savings represents a remarkable return of $5.60 for every dollar spent, without considering the additional gains in worker productivity, reduced absenteeism at work and school, and enhanced quality of life."[102]

The almanac goes on to state that the World Health Organization, Southern Australian Workplace Physical Activity Kit, reports that, "Workplace physical activity programs can reduce sick leave by up to 32 percent and increase productivity by

"Up to 2.7 million lives could be saved annually with sufficient fruit and vegetable intake."

"Low fruit and vegetable intake is among the top 10 selected risk factors for global mortality."

World Health Organization Global Strategy on Diet, Physical Activity and Health. Promoting fruit and vegetable consumption around the world. 2010 up to 52 percent."[103]

"Workplace physical activity programs can reduce sick leave by up to 32 percent and increase productivity by up to 52 percent."[103]

The Canada Life Corporation in Toronto, Canada reports that for every dollar they invested in physical activity programs they showed a return of $3.40 through reduced employee turnover, increased productivity, and decreased medical claims.

There are over 600 studies providing evidence for the health benefits and cost-effectiveness of employee wellness programs. In one review of 32 studies it was found that corporate wellness programs reduced claim costs by 27.8 percent, reduced physician visits by 16.5 percent, reduced hospital admissions by 62.5 percent, reduced disability costs by 34.4 percent and reduced incidence of injury by 24.8 percent. A 1996 study at Providence General Hospital found that a simple workplace wellness program saved 33.6 percent on per person healthcare costs, reduced sick leave by 22.2 percent, reduced Worker's Compensation costs by 83.4 percent and provided a $4.24 return for every dollar invested.[104]

"I don't go around measuring cholesterol. I ask patients what they are eating, what they are doing, how they are living. Lifestyle is much more important than any of these measurements. Now, I have lots of patients who had positive exercise tests, angina, and they are now pain-free, normal exercise tests, no pill."

Dr. Colin Rose - Cardiologist - Faculty, McGill University in Heart of the Matter, CBC Radio - Ideas http://www.cbc.ca/ideas/IDEAS-Catalog.pdf

The amount of evidence for lifestyle intervention is so overwhelming that, once you are aware of it, the fact that it has not become the foundation of healthcare reform becomes incredulous. I believe there can only be two logical explanations. One, people within the Sickness & Treatment Paradigm are so entrenched in this paradigm that they simply are unaware of the evidence for lifestyle intervention. I think this

Why has lifestyle intervention not become part of mainstream healthcare?

is true for some, especially practitioners who get most of their continuing education from pharmaceutical representatives or at pharmaceutical company sponsored seminars. These people are also often instilled with a strong dogmatic bias against intervention that is not based on drugs and surgery. They get indoctrinated very early on in medical education regarding an assumed inherent superiority of the medical system and often develop the highly unscientific stance that drugs and surgery represent the most, if not the only, evidence-based interventions. Pharmaceutical companies obviously have a vested interest in perpetuating this bias and spend billions of dollars doing just this via marketing to practitioners, the public, and policy makers.

How much do medical and other traditionally educated practitioners know about lifestyle? Do they have expertise in this area? Is it part of their education?

This brings us to the second logical explanation, which is that those who profit most from drugs and surgery are highly resistant to changing to a system that significantly reduces their use (sales). The fact that we must all face is that what this information really means is that the practitioners we have come to count on for health advice are uneducated, untrained, and ill equipped when it comes to wellness and prevention. They are undeniably highly trained experts in the practice of diagnosis of disease and the prescription of drugs and surgeries. This is not debatable or in question. What is in question is why this is the only system, and why this system is still being championed as the solution for the chronic illness pandemic or wellness and prevention in general.

The indisputable fact is that the single greatest need in terms of the health of our population and thus our healthcare system is no longer drugs and surgery.

When infectious disease was our greatest threat things were different. However, times have changed and if we don't change our healthcare system to meet these demands we are, without debate, going to be bankrupt in terms of both health and economy. We are trying to fight chronic illness utilizing a paradigm and intervention strategies set up for fighting infectious disease. Chronic illness is not caught or contagious or transmitted; chronic illness is developed over time as the result of chronic lifestyle and environmental stressors. The problem is that we have become so entrenched in the diagnose and fight disease mantra that developed during the era of success with identifying infectious disease agents, and we have developed such a huge industrial machine regarding drugs and surgery, that it has become incredibly difficult to change direction.

Ironically, despite so much information and claims to the contrary, even the solution to the infectious disease epidemics was not solved by the Sickness & Treatment Paradigm methods of diagnosing and treating disease with drugs. It was, in fact, solved by changing the environment. As Dr. Debra Davis PhD, MPH, Professor of Epidemiology and Director of the Center for Environmental Oncology at the University of Pittsburgh Cancer Institute points out in her book, The Secret History of the War on Cancer, "In fact, the decline of epidemics in the nineteenth century had nothing to do with breathtaking scientific advances; all of these came much later."

"Deaths from germ-fed contagious diseases began to ebb long before microscopes or drugs could find or kill them," wrote Dr. Davis, adding, "This decline happened because dirty water, crowded housing, rotten food and dangerous jobs became much less common in developed nations."

What was responsible for the rapid decrease in contagious diseases in early industrial cities: lifestyle and environment changes, or medical intervention?

How sad that our approach to fight these same issues in undeveloped countries has come to be centered around drugs instead of making the living environments of these people healthier. There is no doubt drugs can save a life in a crisis but the real need is to provide clean water, healthy food, safe housing, and safe jobs for these poor people. Only when we do this will they get and stay well. The drugs don't get them well; they simply make them more comfortable on the iceberg or in the pool with a backpack full of rocks. At the end of the day what is the long term benefit of providing poor, starving, disenfranchised, homeless, sick people with drugs UNLESS the causal lifestyle and environmental issues are addressed. The exact same question must be asked regarding the effectiveness of providing over fed, underexercised, comfortably housed, sick people drugs and failing to address the causal lifestyle and environmental issues.

Chapter 9
Finding the Right Paradigm for the Job: Fire Departments or Contractors?

"Learning what to choose, and how to choose, may be the most important education you will ever receive."

Shad Helmstetter

Healthcare has lost its way on so many levels. In every healthcare field whether it be medicine, chiropractic, naturopathy, homeopathy or osteopathy we have become so entrenched in the Sickness & Treatment Paradigm that 'correct' diagnosis and treatment has become more important than patient outcomes. As an intern in any one of the healthcare professions you can get an A+ grade even if all your patients get sicker or die. The whole system has become doctor centered and diagnosis and treatment centered instead of patient centered and outcome centered. As long as you write down what is considered the correct diagnosis and provide what is considered the correct treatment you are considered a good practitioner in this paradigm – the outcomes for the patients are irrelevant with regard to evaluating the worth of the practitioner or intervention. Why? Because it is assumed that if what you do does not help then nothing will. You are not taught to question the accepted intervention even if it doesn't work. If you believe the patient is sick due to bad genes or pathological cell function, then you just believe the reason they are sick and don't get well is due to the inherent weakness of the patient rather than the inherent weakness of the intervention. In fact, you are highly discouraged from questioning accepted interventions or the actions of your peers.

This is not only a significant obstacle to change in terms of the interventions offered, it is a significant obstacle to improving patient outcomes. Let's think about prognosis for a moment. What does a medical prognosis indicate, or, more, importantly, how is it interpreted by doctor and patient? A prognosis is interpreted as the most likely outcome for the patient. How is prognosis determined? Prognosis is determined by looking at outcomes of previous patients with the same diagnosis, who received the same advice and treatment. So what this means is that the doctor and patient expect the prognosis to predict the outcome. If previous patients did not get and stay well neither doctor nor patient expect any different.

The problem is that this is all based on the a priori assumption that the treatment was evidence-based and that is was the best, or only, available treatment option. What arrogance by the practitioner and what hopelessness for the patient. The fact is that the ONLY valid information that can be derived from prognosis is that if you do exactly what the other patients do you will get the same result they did. In other words, if you have a lifestyle caused illness and choose to treat this with drugs and or surgery while never addressing the lifestyle cause, you will have the same prognosis and outcome as everyone else who applied this strategy. My advice? If you don't want the same result don't do the same thing!

How is prognosis determined?

Does this mean that there is no need or benefit for drugs and surgery or for the Sickness & Treatment Paradigm or the practitioners that work within it? Of course not. The fact that drugs and surgery are not viable options for wellness and prevention certainly does not determine whether or not they are viable options for those times and those patients that require such an intervention in a crisis or for palliating symptoms. However, and this is extremely important, we MUST not make the absurd assumption that if wellness and prevention interventions are not viable options for crisis intervention or instantly palliating symptoms, that they are not viable options for improving health and preventing illness.

The Fire Department Analogy

I want you to understand how it is possible for the Sickness & Treatment Paradigm, for drugs and surgery, to be able to save a life in a crisis, but not be appropriate for wellness and prevention and vice versa. I also want to elucidate the differences between these approaches so that you can determine when one, the other, or both are appropriate.

For this analogy your mind and body are your house, medical doctors are the fire department, and lifestyle practitioners are the contractors - the house maintenance and renovation experts. Now, imagine your house is on fire. It is an emergency. Who should you call, the fire department or the renovation and maintenance experts?

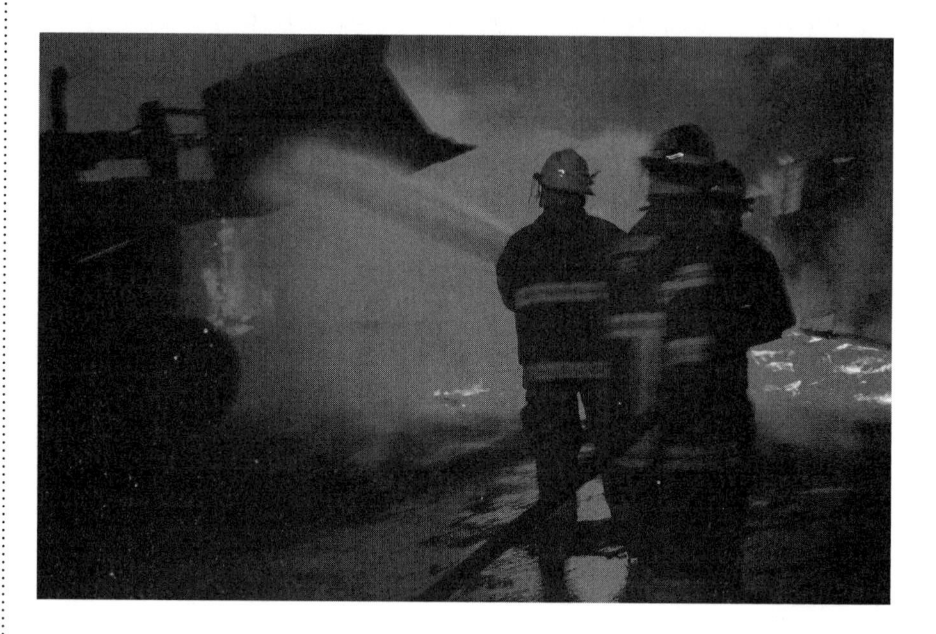

Would it be logical to call the fire department to use their axes and fire hoses to get and keep your house well?

I hope you said the fire department. Now, what will the fire department do when they get to your burning house? Well, what they do will depend on what tools they have to work with. What tools does the fire department have? The tools that they have developed are congruent with their goal to put out fires (treat disease risk factors and symptoms). They have axes and fire hoses (drugs and surgery). What will they use these for? They will use the axes to break out all your windows, chop down your door, and chop open your walls. They will use the hoses to soak all the walls and furnishings of your home.

What is the result? If you are lucky, if they get there in time and do not make any big mistakes, they will save the life of your house. For this you should be eternally grateful. Now, what is left after they have put out the fire? A huge mess to clean up. In fact, your house is now in far worse shape than it was before the fire ever started. Think about it, what would happen if you did not have a fire but decided to use axes and fire hoses on your house? Would this not do damage to your house? Of course it would. Now, think about drugs and surgery for a second. What happens if you give a healthy person drugs or surgery? Do drugs and surgery not leave a mess, do they not damage the cells of the body and make your house less healthy? Of course they do.

So now what will you do? Who will you call to restore your house back to health, back to the state it was in before the fire (or perhaps even better shape if your house was not well maintained at the time of the fire)? Would you think it logical to call back the fire department? Do you think more axes and fire hoses could ever restore your house to proper function? Of course not, that is an absurd notion. Not as absurd as the fire department claiming that they could do this, or that nobody else could, but nonetheless still very absurd.

So who should you call? The restoration and maintenance experts, people with the tools and knowledge regarding what materials are needed to restore your house to working order. What tools would such experts have? Hammers, nails, paint, wiring, wood, and any other materials that the blueprint of the house indicated were required. The tools they have are all congruent with their goal to restore and maintain the function of your house; they are the ingredients that your house needs for healthy function.

Would you call restoration and maintenance contractors to put out your house fire?

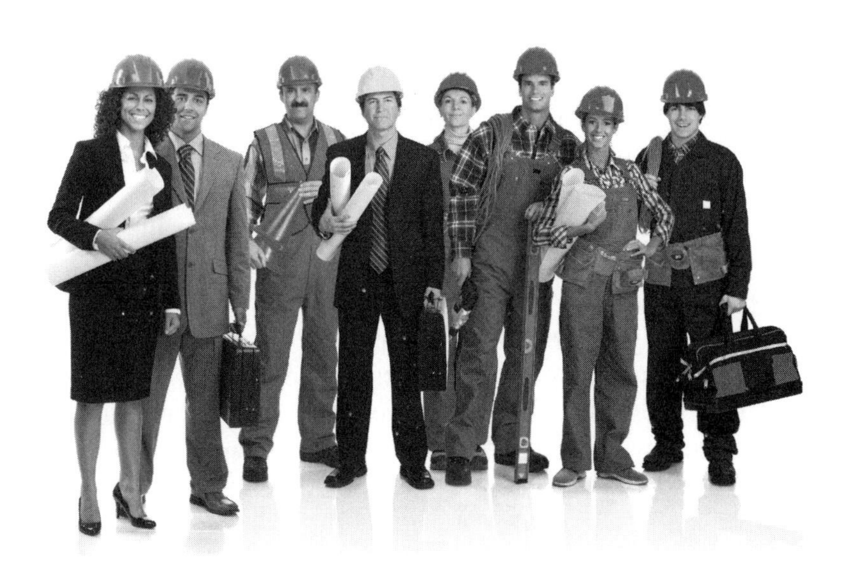

Now imagine if the fire department convinced everyone, including themselves, to judge the worth of the restoration and maintenance experts according to the ability to put out fires or their legal ability to use axes and fire hoses. Obviously, the restoration and maintenance experts would look pretty incompetent trying to put out a fire with paint brushes and hammers. The fire department could, with scientific accuracy, tell everyone how incompetent the restoration and maintenance experts are at putting out fires. In fact, the fire department could demand scientific evidence from the restoration and maintenance experts to show that they could put out fires, and no matter how hard they tried, the restoration and maintenance experts would never be able to show they were competent at putting out fires.

Would axes and fire hoses be logical tools to prevent house fires?

But wait a minute, I hope you are thinking. What if the worth of the fire department was assessed by how well they could restore and maintain a house? They would look as incompetent at this as the restoration and maintenance workers would at putting out a fire. Could you imagine the fire department showing up with axes and fire hoses and claiming they could improve the health and function of the house? How absurd. Science would show that no matter how often the fire department used axes and fire hoses, no matter how much technology they had to make new axes and fire hoses, they would always be totally incompetent in terms of improving the health and function of houses. What about preventing fires? Do you think showing up at a fire with axes and fire hoses could ever prevent a fire? Of course not. But what if they got amazing technology to detect a fire earlier and earlier so they could break down the doors and spray the house earlier and earlier, would this ever prevent a fire?

So, who is the better expert, who is more valid, who are 'real house doctors' and who are the 'quack' house doctors? Both are valid experts and real doctors and neither are quacks if you assess them within their own paradigms, within their own areas of expertise. The trick is to use these experts and their interventions at the appropriate times. The fire department should be a last resort and only used when there is a fire. The goal should be to NEVER need the fire department. The restoration and maintenance experts should be the last resort for a fire and the first and only resort for getting and keeping your house well. The goal should be to ALWAYS utilize them regularly or, even better, to get them to teach you how to take care of your own house.

But what about all the fire department studies showing that they prevent fires? Well, think about it for a second. If you randomly assigned 50,000 houses to each group in a randomized controlled trial and one group you sprayed down once a week with water and the other group you sprayed down once a week with placebo water (air), what would the results be?

Well it depends on which questions you ask, doesn't it? The fire department only asks fire-related or fire symptom-related questions. In this case the fire department scientists would ask if spraying down the houses resulted in a statistically significant reduction in fires or fire symptoms (smoke, heat, fire alarms going off, etc). Good news - regularly spraying down houses with water results in significantly less fires and symptoms of fires. Armed with this scientific evidence from the gold standard RCT clinical trial, the fire department could then recommend regularly spraying down houses and claim that it prevents fires or symptoms of fires.

Would more fire departments and/or more axes and fire hoses ever result in healthier houses?

Are you thinking what I'm thinking? Wouldn't regularly spraying down houses with water cause them to rot? Yes it would, that is called a side effect. This does not, however, erase the fact that these houses were saved from the ravages of fire. Luckily, the fire department studies do not ask whether or not regularly spraying down the houses is healthy; they only ask if it can reduce fires and symptoms of fires. They also don't ask if the houses that do not get sprayed down and do not burn down live longer, happier lives. Why would they? They don't even ask if the houses that do get sprayed down live longer, happier lives. These are not fire department-related questions. Most importantly the fire department NEVER compares regular intervention from the renovation and maintenance interventions to the regular water spraying with respect to house longevity or house health and function.

The restoration and maintenance scientists, of which there are very few because all the schools are either run or controlled by the fire department and the suppliers of axes and hoses, are busy trying to point out the futility of this approach. In fact, the restoration and maintenance scientists have shown beyond a reasonable doubt that for the last 50 years - even though there have been more firefighters, more fire trucks, more fire stations, and more axes and hoses every year – (more doctors, nurses, hospitals, drugs and surgeries) there have also been more sick and dying houses each year for the past

50 years.

The fire department just responds that they need more money for more fire fighters, more fire trucks, more fire stations, and more axes and hoses. The advertising and lobbyist budget for the fire department, which comes from the makers of axes and hoses, is so huge that they have actually convinced politicians and voters that this is the only scientific approach. In fact, say the fire department and axes and fire hose scientists, the restoration and maintenance experts can't even put out fires so their opinions are irrelevant. They are not even allowed to use axes and fire hoses, they are not even real house doctors, they are axe-free practitioners.

Does being a firefighter and being an expert in putting out fires automatically make you an expert in house renovation and maintenance?

The restoration and maintenance workers argue that they do not want to put out house fires. Their outcome goals are to restore and maintain the health and function of the houses and to prevent fires and other preventable house damage. They want to improve the quality and quantity of the lives of houses. They contend that this is the only sane way to approach the health of houses. They also contend that the fire department is a very important service to have, but that to organize the entire house health system around the concept of fire is unscientific, illogical, and impotent. They point out that detecting and putting out fires can never prevent a fire.

The fire department and axe manufacturers just repeat that they have scientific studies to show they can put out fires and prevent fires and symptoms of fires with the regular use of axes and fire hoses. They also repeat that the restoration and maintenance experts can't do this. They constantly evoke fear by repeatedly pointing out how horrible fires are and how frequent they are and how all citizens must work together to try and find the very best treatments for fires.

The restoration and maintenance experts repeat that putting out fires and treating the symptoms of fires does not improve the health of houses. They also point out that the root cause of fires is not a lack of, or deficiency in, axes or fire hoses. They also point out that houses don't spontaneously combust – the fire department argues that they do, that fires are genetic.

The argument continues but the fire department controls all the resources and schools, has all the money for marketing, has government support for coverage for axes and fire hoses, and has thousands and thousands of research scientists proving that axes and fire hoses can put out fires. All the restoration and maintenance department has is unequivocal evidence that axes and fire hoses have never been, and will never be, valid solutions to get and keep houses well or to prevent fires. All the restoration and maintenance department has is unequivocal evidence that their interventions are valid solutions to get and keep houses well and to prevent fires. The question being begged is, why does the fire department still have all the resources and government support? Paradigm and profit.

Okay, you are thinking, "I get it, but my house health insurance only covers axes and fire hoses." Of course it does; insurance is for emergencies, not for restoration and maintenance. Does your car insurance cover oil changes and tune-ups? Does your house insurance cover painting and eaves cleaning? Does your life insurance cover going to the gym or eating healthy food? Restoration and maintenance is not an insurance issue, it is a lifestyle and common sense issue. Emergency or accident insurance does not cover wellness and prevention expenses. However, what is happening now is that health insurance, and the corporations who pay for it, are beginning to see the huge return on investment of covering wellness and prevention. This is why there are so many workplace wellness programs now and why I got invited to give the keynote address at a health insurance convention.

Is it possible to reduce symptoms or risk factors with a drug and not increase health? What happens if we define the success of an intervention by changes in symptoms and/or risk factors instead of changes in health and function?

Drugs and surgery will always have a place in crisis intervention and symptom reduction, and when used appropriately they can save lives and alleviate suffering. These are the aims of the Sickness & Treatment Paradigm interventions and research and they have developed many useful ways to prevent death in acute crisis and to make unhealthy people feel better. We should all be grateful for the advances in these areas.

However, the Sickness & Treatment Paradigm interventions were never designed to improve health and function. This is not the aim of Sickness & Treatment Paradigm intervention or research. They have not developed any tools to improve or restore cell function and health; this is outside the scope of Sickness & Treatment Paradigm education and practice. Sickness & Treatment Paradigm interventions do not produce health. Sickness & Treatment Paradigm care is sickness care, not health care. Understanding this can literally save your life.

At the core of the Sickness & Treatment Paradigm is the belief that cell function is solely under genetic control and that genes inherently make mistakes that result in errors in cell function. Sickness & Treatment Paradigm scientists and practitioners choose to over-ride the ability of the genes to control and regulate the body. The Sickness & Treatment Paradigm includes the belief that the intelligence of the genetic code is simply inherently prone to failures. The goal of Sickness & Treatment Paradigm research and intervention is to reduce symptoms or treat diseases that they believe result from the inherent failures of the genes to properly control and regulate the body.

If health is the genetic expression of environment, what should be the focus of interventions aimed at getting and keeping patients well?

Sickness & Treatment Paradigm science and scope of practice does not include the concept of human ecosystem health and function. Sickness & Treatment Paradigm scientists and practitioners consider a reduction in symptoms or risk factors a successful result, regardless of whether or not the health and function status of the patient has been improved. An example would be to lower blood pressure or cholesterol or pain with a drug or therapy while disregarding the fact that this not only does not increase the health of the patient, it very often decreases it. Sickness & Treatment Paradigm scientists and practitioners do not attempt to measure lifestyle or health and function because it is not these concepts which drive the research questions and clinical outcome goals of the Sickness & Treatment Paradigm.

The Wellness & Prevention Paradigm is founded on the knowledge that the innate genetic intelligence is sound and that the natural expression of this intelligence is a state of physiology that is best suited to survive and/or thrive in any given environment.

Wellness & Prevention Paradigm scientists and practitioners recognize the fact that the environment determines the physiology that the innate genetic intelligence will express. Physiology is the genetic (or epigenetic) expression of the environment. Thus the goal of Wellness & Prevention Paradigm research and intervention is to identify and provide genetically congruent environments and genetically congruent lifestyle behaviors.

Wellness & Prevention Paradigm science and scope of practice do not include the concepts of symptom and disease treatment or therapy. Wellness & Prevention Paradigm scientists and practitioners consider an improvement in human ecosystem health and function a successful result. Symptoms are seen as signals that the ecosystem is under stress and crying out for appropriate environmental changes. Removing the ability of the body to send these signals and failing to address the underlying causes is illogical within the Wellness & Prevention Paradigm.

Wellness & Prevention Paradigm researchers and clinicians do not attempt to diagnose and treat disease risk factors or symptoms because it is not these concepts which drive the research questions and clinical outcome goals of the Wellness & Prevention Paradigm. Symptoms and disease are not present in states of healthy function, so as healthy function is restored symptoms naturally fade away. Importantly however, symptoms and signs of disease can be absent even during states of adaptive cell function and for this reason the indicator for the need for Wellness & Prevention Paradigm intervention is not signs and symptoms of disease but an assessment of environment, lifestyle, and states of health and function.

If your oil light came on would it be logical to pay a mechanic to cut the wire to make it go off? If your smoke detector was sounding alarm would it be logical to remove the batteries?

The aim of prescription drugs is over ride our ability to adapt to or physiologically express our environment. Drugs actually block the ability of our genes to adapt our physiology to match environmental demand.

The real problem with this approach is that if you leave the person in the toxic Petri dish or on the iceberg and don't allow them to have the symptoms of living in that toxic Petri dish or on that iceberg, which are all the warning signals and motivators to change environments or lifestyle choices, the people are really just being allowed to commit suicide comfortably. Drugs not only prevent the innate intelligence of our genes from expressing appropriate adaptive physiology to meet environmental demand, they also interfere with the ability for our genes and cells to send us warning signals. It is like cutting the wire to the oil light in your car or removing the batteries in your smoke alarm.

I want you to think about something else. This might help you understand the power of the prescription drug lobby and the power of the belief system about prescription drugs that they have so successfully perpetuated. Do you know that they do not test for prescription drugs when someone has been in a car accident or an accident at work? They will test for alcohol and marijuana and cocaine and heroin and other illegal drugs but they do not test for the EXACT SAME classes of legal prescription drugs. Do you think this is because prescription drugs don't affect the ability to drive or operate machinery the same way illegal drugs do?

Have you ever considered the fact that if you get in an accident and have an open beer bottle in the car you are immediately charged with a crime. Shockingly, you could run over a group of kids and if you have an open prescription bottle in the car or a bloodstream full of prescription drugs when you are tested you are not charged. How can this be? Once again we see the influence of profit and paradigm.

Why don't they test for prescription drugs at car accidents and workplace accidents?

Think about the advertisements for the antacids on television. You get the overweight, chronically ill dude bellying up to the café counter and wondering whether he should order the salad or what he is really craving, the bacon double cheese burger, fries with gravy, and the soda. The problem, he thinks, is that if he eats what he really wants he is going to get indigestion. No problem. In comes the solution – antacids. The announcer tells us that if the dude takes the antacids beforehand he can enjoy the death on a plate meal he really craves. In other words, treat the symptoms, shut off the warning signals and you can commit suicide with your lifestyle choices more comfortably. There are countless ways the Sickness & Treatment Paradigm folks can make you comfortable on the iceberg or in the pool with a big load of rocks in your backpack.

They literally determine whether or not a drug has a good or a bad effect, not by whether or not it makes the person healthier, but by whether or not it can turn off the symptoms or change a risk factor.

Drugs aren't evaluated for effectiveness based on their ability to produce health or function. They're evaluated based on whether or not they can shut off symptoms.

This is actually harming you because symptoms are your body's way of saying how you're eating, moving and thinking, the environment that you are living in, is toxic and deficient, that your cells need help and that you need to make changes. Certainly symptom relief can be very appropriate IF the lifestyle causes are being addressed and IF everyone is aware that symptom status is an invalid way to determine health status. If people think they are getting healthier by taking drugs to decrease symptoms or change risk factors they are wrong – just ask the insurance actuaries.

Let's think about what happens in a hospital for a second. How many of you think that you could develop a better diet plan than what is in your local hospital? And we've got people with tubes hanging out of them, and we've got seven people making sure they get the right pill, and then they serve them a pork chop with powdered gravy and ice cream – because there's no connection being made between how these people are eating and their health or ability to recover. The focus is not on restoring healthy cell function, the focus is on treating symptoms and changing disease risk factors. I can understand and empathize and even agree with it if the situation is an acute emergency. I just want everyone to understand that no matter what state of health we are in, if we want our cells to function better, if we want to increase our state of health and function, the only way to do this is to provide our cells with what they need and avoid those things which are toxic.

Is the food served in hospitals, the food served to our sickest citizens, healthy?

The only way to solve a problem caused by toxicity and deficiency is to remove the toxicity or add the essential ingredient that you're deficient in. That's it. We have an entire system that we call healthcare, which has nothing to do with either of these things. This is the crux of the problem.

That doesn't mean to say they are not phenomenal at sometimes stopping us from shooting toward death. And we should all be grateful for those things. I am. Medicine has saved my life in an acute emergency, and I am eternally grateful for that. However the truth of the matter is, as difficult as it might be to admit, that there is nothing in drugs or surgery that is going to produce healthy cells and there's nothing in drugs or surgery that is going to prevent the need for drugs or surgery.

A few years ago I went to see a friend of mine who was diagnosed with cancer. I had not been in a hospital for a long time, probably 15 years earlier when I last had to go and get stitched up after a rugby game. The first thing I saw when I went in the hospital was, "Thank you for the $7 Million." I thought to myself wow, after all the tax money they still needed another $7 million dollars for treating sickness in this place. I went around the corner, and there was a person in a wheelchair with a urine bag on the side of it, with a coffee and a donut – in the hospital! I thought to myself, how can we have a donut shop in a hospital and call that sane? I also thought about how nobody wants to be in a hospital yet they are overflowing. How sad. I also thought how sad it was that 80 percent of the people were there for preventable reasons, for reasons that were avoidable with healthier lifestyle habits.

What percentage of the people in your local hospital are there due to lifestyle - due to preventable illness? How many of them or their doctors recognize this fact?

They diagnosed and treated my friend's cancer and they bought him some survival time; they bought him some time to change his environment and his lifestyle choices. Thank goodness this service was available and damn the fact that it is needed so often for preventable illnesses. I remember I bought him a special blender that can chop anything and it is great for making fruit and vegetable smoothies. I'll never forget when I dropped it off at his house. The whole house was filled with gifts from people, mostly cakes and cookies and that kind of thing. I just kept thinking how unhealthy all that was and how far removed we are from reality that we can, out of sincere love, give junk-food to a person with cancer. I wanted to take it all away. I didn't say anything. I felt like a coward afterward. I didn't want to offend anyone yet I cared so deeply for my friend. It is one of the few times in my life that I have just sat down and wept.

Most people just would never make a connection between junk-food and lowered immunity, higher insulin, decreased sex hormone binding globulin, increased inflammation, and more stress hormones. They just think of it as a harmless treat that might have a few extra calories which certainly is not an issue for someone who has lost so much weight from cancer or cancer treatment. These are not bad people with anything other than loving intention. I am not criticizing or blaming anybody; I'm trying to save lives. I just need you and everyone else to understand that there are no consequence-free choices. Every meal either pushes you toward health or away. We need to be extra vigilant about this when we are sick, not less.

I often think to myself that the marketing is so successful

now that people think that they are depriving themselves, their friends, or their children if they don't feed them junk-food. That's how successful the marketing is. If we send our children to school overweight, or with acne, or with weakened immunity whose fault is that? It isn't our children's fault. How can we possibly use the excuse that they won't eat anything else? When I hear this I always say, "ya, I know what you mean, my kids just won't stop smoking cigars and drinking wine at dinner." People look at me like I am crazy, which I would be if I allowed my children to choose such behaviors. But would I be sane if I let them refuse to eat vegetables and fruits and healthy food and instead gave them the processed, calorie-rich, nutrient-poor, chemically-filled food they ask for (often because their friends are getting it), let them sit on the couch watching television or playing video games, and neglected to consciously fill them with love and attention and self-esteem?

Give me a break - be the parent. I ask my kids if they want me to be a good daddy or a bad daddy. I tell them I could leave them alone in the house, I could forget to give them enough blankets, I could stop telling them how much I love them and how proud of them I am every day, I could do a lot of bad things if they preferred it. They always say they want me to be a good daddy. Then I ask them, "does a good daddy make sure his children eat foods to make them healthy, strong, and smart or does a good daddy let his kids eat foods that are going to make them unhealthy, weak, and slow?" Kids are smart, tell them the truth, tell them why you make the decisions you do.

How did we get convinced that giving a child junk-food is a treat and an act of affection rather than an act of cruelty?

Giving children or anyone else foods that are toxic is not being more loving or being a better friend or parent. You are marketed to believe it is more loving, but it is just poisoning people you love or poisoning yourself. You are far too important and so are your children for me to allow you to poison yourselves without telling you the truth. Now a home-made dessert, without any chemicals or trans fats or hydrogenated fats, once or twice a week is not what I am discussing here. I am talking about the processed foods, the breakfast cereals, the packaged lunch stuff that is made in a chemical factory rather than grown on a farm.

People always ask me, "Dr. Chestnut can you teach me how to read a food label?" I always respond the same way. "If it has a label on it, it is not food." If all you did was change your diet to exclude anything with a label you would be well on your way to better health.

The marketing is so successful that Wellness & Prevention Paradigm parents are the outliers in society. We are seen as quack-like or obsessive because we don't want our kids to eat unhealthy foods. You know the line, 'everything in moderation'. As my colleague Dr. Baxter brilliantly says, the moderation argument only makes sense if you are willing to accept moderate amounts of health, to express a moderate amount of your potential for happiness and vitality, and to chronically suffer with moderate amounts of disease.

When people say, "everything in moderation" do they mean they want to express only moderate amounts of health and to chronically suffer with moderate amounts of sickness?

Do the Sickness & Treatment Paradigm parents have any actual evidence that their kids are unaffected by these foods or that feeding their children a healthier diet would not greatly benefit their children? Of course not. It is because the marketing campaigns are so successful that these parents just assume that the foods sold in supermarkets or fed for school lunches could not possibly be pushing their children to cancer, diabetes, obesity, ADHD, infertility, dementia, and heart disease. What do they think is responsible for the exponential rise in chronic illness? Oh ya, bad genes, bad cells, or bad luck. They also have their 'health experts', their Sickness & Treatment Paradigm practitioners, to confirm this belief.

I can't tell you how many kids I have seen clinically that are literally junk-food junkies and have been prescribed course after course of antibiotics and steroid creams and Ritalin and asthma and allergy medications. Parents bring me these kids in desperation or after they hear I have helped another child. They come in expecting me to tell them that I have some special 'treatment' or 'magic bullet', or specific 'natural' cure for the illness or symptoms their child is suffering with. The first thing I tell them is that there are no such things. The ONLY thing to do is to change their lifestyle patterns, to remove the toxins they are putting into their bodies and to fill their bodies up with the nutrients, movement and exercise stimulation, and self confidence and love and social connections they genetically require. I don't provide lifestyle recommendations based on treating disease. I make lifestyle recommendations based on the species wide genetic requirements for human beings. I simply teach them how to eat, how to move, and how to think and interact in ways that are sufficient and pure, in ways that are genetically congruent and then I sit back and watch as their ecosystems recover and their health and lives significantly improve.

Their Sickness & Treatment Paradigm practitioners just ignore all this stuff; for the life of me I cannot understand why we would think it sane or ethical to fill these children with drugs before we addressed lifestyle.

Of course that is because I view things through a different paradigm. I hope you are starting to do the same. Thankfully more and people are becoming aware of this. An easy to read, incredibly well referenced book on the topic is *Anticancer – A New Way of Life* written by David Servan-Schreiber. Dr. Schreiber is an M.D., Ph.D. neuroscientist who developed a brain tumor. He wrote his book in response to his experience, particularly with respect to the advice, or lack of advice, he was given by his oncologist regarding the importance of lifestyle. When he asked his oncologist, whom he describes as a leading light of modern medicine, what lifestyle choices he should be making the answer he got shocked him. His oncologist told him that lifestyle was irrelevant, that all that all they could do was conduct regular screenings to see if his cancer came back so they could treat it as early as possible.

Is expertise in diagnosis and treatment applicable to issues of wellness and prevention? Are opinions of diagnosis and treatment experts regarding wellness and prevention valid?

Leading lights within the Sickness & Treatment Paradigm are leading lights in diagnosis and treatment of disease, not wellness and prevention. They are fire department experts, not house maintenance experts. I have no issue with this, I am grateful for these hard working, intelligent, caring practitioners. The problem is that this leading light of modern medicine, this very influential practitioner whose words would have been followed like gospel by most, did not refer his patient to a leading light in the Wellness & Prevention Paradigm, admit he was too ignorant of the available literature to provide an informed opinion, or suggest that the patient should seek their own information.

This person with NO EXPERTISE but with HUGE INFLUENCE gave advice that was not only uninformed, it was incorrect and DEADLY. His expertise and clinical prowess in the Sickness & Treatment Paradigm undoubtedly saves lives. How tragic that his advice regarding lifestyle undoubtedly costs lives. There is just no reason for this to be occurring.

Now I don't want there to be ANY confusion about this. I am not suggesting that there is evidence that patients should be referred to Wellness & Prevention Paradigm practitioners for cancer treatment. I am insisting that they should be referred to such practitioners for cancer prevention strategies and for advice about strategies to maximize chances of recovering health and function. Disease treatment is not within the scope of expertise or practice of such practitioners. What I am suggesting, in fact insisting, is that every person who wants to get and stay well should be referred to, or seek out lifestyle advice from, a qualified Wellness & Prevention Paradigm practitioner.

It is not one OR the other, if people are very sick they will most certainly very often require both Sickness & Treatment Paradigm experts AND Wellness & Prevention Paradigm experts.

Are "natural" treatments for disease anymore likely to address the lifestyle causes of illness than drug and surgical treatments?

'Natural' Treatments are just More Treatments

This is probably a good time to point out the fact that the 'natural' disease and symptom treatment industry is now a multi-billion dollar industry. Health food stores stock very few healthy foods and make a very small percentage of their revenue from selling health food. These stores are filled with 'natural' pills, most of them making unsubstantiated, unethical claims regarding the ability to treat symptoms and disease. This is a predatory industry and it takes advantage of the poor people that have already been taken advantage of and let down by the drug industry.

This is VERY important. What determines if an intervention is within the Sickness & Treatment Paradigm or the Wellness & Prevention Paradigm has NOTHING to do with whether said intervention is 'natural', what kind of practitioner prescribed or recommended it, or whether it came from a pharmacy or a health food store or supplement store. I cannot emphasize this point enough to you or the practitioners I teach.

When people are sick they are vulnerable, they want nothing more than to hear about a magic cure, a magical new drug or a magical new herb or plant or botanical or enzyme. These things do not exist.

Health cannot be obtained from the treatment of symptoms or disease regardless of what that treatment is. Therapies, pharmaceuticals and nutraceuticals are all Sickness & Treatment Paradigm interventions. If any intervention is aimed at symptoms or disease, if any intervention is symptom or disease specific, it is NOT a Wellness & Prevention intervention.

Supplement stores and supplement catalogues have hundreds and hundreds of products, they are impossible to differentiate from the pharmacies. These products are all categorized by disease or symptom and are prescribed or recommended based on whether you have the disease or symptom. Do you actually think it matters if the axe and fire hose are from an herb or a chemical factory, from a pharmacy or a health food store? They do the same thing. Sure one might have less side effects but the targeted effects are identical. Do you think these 'natural' treatments get rocks out of your backpack or get you off the iceberg? Do you think they address the symptoms and illnesses you have that are caused by deficiencies in nutrients, a lack of exercise, or a lack of positive thoughts and social interactions? Of course they don't!

How do we differentiate between wellness and prevention, and sickness and treatment, interventions?

How do we determine if an intervention is within the Wellness & Prevention Paradigm? It is very easy. First, ask yourself if the intervention represents a lifestyle change aimed at increasing your health rather than a treatment aimed at a disease symptom or risk factor. Next, ask yourself if this lifestyle recommendation represents adding a genetically required ingredient or raw material. Next, and this one is the best litmus test of all, ask yourself if the recommendation is something that is required for every member of the human species, if it is a species wide requirement. There is no nutrient, no movement or exercise requirement, and no thinking and social interaction requirement that is unique to any member of any species – unless they have a documented genetic variant which is so rare it is hardly worth mentioning. Remember, if you require it, we all require it.

Does this mean that there is never an appropriate time for supplementation? No it does not, however, we must be able to determine which supplements, out of the thousands and thousands that are being marketed and sold, are evidence-based, required, and effective in terms of increasing health and function.

The supplement industry is so predatory and so full of misinformation that I created my own company. When I first created my post-graduate wellness lifestyle certification program for the International Chiropractors Association I was courted by a great many supplement companies and promised all kinds of riches if I took on one of these companies as the official supplement line of the program. I have no issue with making a profit from an ethical service, what I have a problem with is making a profit from taking advantage of sick, vulnerable people. My program was the first in history taught completely within the Wellness & Prevention Paradigm, I'm quite certain it remains the only such program. My research had brought me to the conclusion that there were a few supplements that the human species now requires, the problem was I could not find a single supplement company that operated within the Wellness & Prevention Paradigm. There were companies that offered the supplements that research supported but the problem was they also offered catalogues full of Sickness & Treatment Paradigm 'natural' products aimed at treating disease symptoms and risk factors.

What valid selection criteria should we apply to choosing supplements.

On principle I could not bring myself to become affiliated with these companies. The only solution was to create my own company so this is what I did. I created the first, and ONLY, supplement company that operates exclusively within the Wellness & Prevention Paradigm – Innate Choice™ (www.innatechoice.com). You can go to the website and get FREE information on supplementation, and you can watch FREE information videos. We don't collect your email or any other contact information and we don't require you to purchase anything. We just want you to get the information you need to make an informed, healthy decision about supplementation.

The first thing I did was trademark the slogan, 'Everybody – Everyday – For Life!™' I did this because this is the only type of supplement anyone should ever take – one that is required by everybody (every member of the species), everyday, for life. This criteria immediately filters out any product that is aimed at the treatment of disease. That is the first criteria you should use before deciding to take any supplement for wellness and prevention. The second criteria is that the supplement must represent an ESSENTIAL nutrient. This means it must represent nutrients that your body cannot make itself; it means it must represent a genetically required ingredient or raw material. The third criteria is that you could not get this essential nutrient from a reasonable change to your diet. The best supplement is no supplement, the best way to get essential nutrients is in foods in your diet. The fourth criteria is that there must be a body of evidence supporting the health and function and/or prevention benefits of taking the supplement. This criteria is redundant if you only choose essential nutrients because if the supplement represents a scientifically established essential nutrient then there is, by definition, already a body of evidence regarding the importance of this nutrient for the human species.

Still, I like to put this in to encourage everyone to apply the same standard of evidence to 'natural' products as pharmaceutical ones. Often companies get a miss on providing any evidence simply because they claim their products are 'natural'. Be aware of this.

The fifth criteria is that the supplement should fully disclose all ingredients and third party testing results. The sixth criteria is that the supplement should be in the most naturally occurring form possible, it should be altered as little as possible, it should be in whole food form not isolated individual nutrients, it should be in the same biochemical form as found in nature. Humans have never, and will never improve upon nature. Our genes evolved or were created synergistically with foods and nutrients as they are found in nature. I will provide the details of the supplements that meet these criteria in the final chapter where I leave you with some lifestyle recommendations.

Have humans ever improved nature or a natural ecosystem?

Chapter 10
Wellness and Prevention: 21st Century Healthcare

"To administer medicines to diseases that have already developed and to suppress revolts which have already begun is comparable to the behavior of those persons who begin to dig a well after they have become thirsty, and of those who begin to cast weapons after they have already engaged in battle. Would these actions not be too late?"

The Yellow Emperor's Classic of Internal Medicine, 200 BC

We need a completely new system based on a completely new paradigm. We need a healthcare system that is based on determining why we get sick and how we can get and stay well. We need a system that addresses the cause of illness and provides the required resources to get and stay well. We don't need to reform a system based on an incorrect paradigm. We can't get a solution by reforming how we ask and answer the wrong questions. We need a new paradigm, we need the Wellness & Prevention Paradigm and the lifestyle-centric research and clinical interventions that arise from it.

There can be no debate regarding the fact that lifestyle intervention must become the foundation of healthcare reform.

We don't need a more efficient system of treating the effects of poor lifestyle with drugs and surgery. Offering drugs and surgery as the solution for chronic illness prevention or cure is illogical, unscientific, and hopeless. The only solution with any hope, that is evidence-based, and that is at all logical, is lifestyle intervention.

What this means, just so there is no confusion, is that your hope, your future, and your health destiny, are your responsibility. It is YOUR choices that will make the greatest difference. Lifestyle centric practitioners operating within the Wellness & Prevention Paradigm can help you discover which choices you should make and the best ones will even offer advice and programs to empower you to make these choices. However, in the end, regardless of any practitioner or intervention you utilize, it will be your knowledge, your beliefs, and your actions that will determine your health, vitality and longevity more than anything else.

What we need now are Wellness & Prevention Paradigm practitioners who have the knowledge and skills to teach, inspire, empower, coach, and role model healthy lifestyle change.

We need an entirely new breed of healthcare professionals, we need an entirely new healthcare field. We need lifestyle practitioners practicing within the field of wellness and prevention. We need to think outside the current sickness and treatment box and start thinking within the Wellness & Prevention Paradigm. We need to stop categorizing practitioners by profession and start categorizing practitioners by their knowledge and by their ability to elicit lifestyle change.

If healthy lifestyle behaviors are the solution to get and stay well, what variables determine effectiveness of care?

Who cares what letters a practitioner has after her or his name if she or he cannot increase the health of patients? If we admit that the only solution is lifestyle change then we must also admit that the only valid way to measure the effectiveness of a lifestyle intervention, or of a lifestyle practitioner, is by the actual patient lifestyle changes and subsequent health changes that are elicited. Patient behavior choice is the key to wellness and prevention and thus empowering patients to make healthy choices is the foundation of wellness and prevention practice.

This changes EVERYTHING. The entire Sickness & Treatment Paradigm is based on specific diagnosis to determine a specific drug or surgical treatment. Diagnosis of disease is not relevant when it comes to determining which lifestyle behaviors are required for wellness and prevention. If you can diagnose it you cannot, by definition, prevent it because it is already present. Lifestyle patterns - lifestyle choices and living environments - are the outcome goals and the variables that must be measured and documented. Because both stressors and the genetically required ingredients or raw materials for the expression of health are SPECIES WIDE, each member of the species, each patient, requires the same eating, moving, thinking, and social interaction patterns to be well.

Think about it. Does it matter what diagnosis you have, or should every human, regardless of diagnosis, eat healthy foods, exercise, and think and interact positively? Of course they should. Would every human, regardless of diagnosis, benefit from eating healthier foods, more healthy exercise (within their abilities of course), and more healthy thought and social interaction patterns? Of course they would. This is very obvious in the lifestyle literature. Even when the people providing the intervention have no information regarding the disease status of the subjects the interventions still improve the health of the subjects.

In fact, what is very interesting, is that you can put a group of people with a huge variety of different diagnoses, risk factors and symptoms into an exercise class, onto a healthier diet, or into a program of relaxation and stress reduction and they ALL get better! Lifestyle is a true panacea, not for treating disease, but for improving health.

Is a disease diagnosis required to determine if someone requires lifestyle intervention?

You will begin to understand that there are panaceas. Panaceas are simply those things that we genetically require and are missing or are deficient in. If everyone is suffering from a deficiency of vitamin C then vitamin C is a panacea for improving cell function in this population. Now imagine if, like me, you spent your life studying what the human species requires in terms of raw materials from the environment with respect to eating, moving, thinking, and interacting. Imagine if your mission was to create a healthcare system that trained doctors to determine whether or not patients were sufficient in what they genetically require or if they were toxic with things that were genetically incongruent and then teach them how to address these causal issues? This is exactly what I have taught to over 5000 doctors in my Wellness Lifestyle Certification Program. The results have been extraordinary.

How great it will be when the Wellness & Prevention Paradigm is the foundation of healthcare and so much of the tragic suffering and death are prevented. This is not a pipe dream. This is an evidence-based goal and it is an achievable goal.

It is not a lack of evidence that has prevented this goal from being achieved, it is the lack of implementation of the evidence into practice. It is a lack of dissemination of this evidence to, and the acceptance of this evidence by, practitioners, citizens, corporations, and policy makers. It is a lack of asking and accurately answering the two most important questions – why are we sick and what is required to get and stay well. It is a lack of viewing human health and sickness within the Wellness & Prevention Paradigm.

I have devoted my professional life to creating a shift to the Wellness & Prevention Paradigm. I have taught thousands and thousands of chiropractors and other practitioners and healthcare employees. I created, and wrote the four textbooks, for my post-graduate Wellness Lifestyle Certification Program over five years ago. I will always be grateful to the International Chiropractors Association for being so progressive and supporting my mission to create credentialed wellness and prevention experts. This program was, and remains, revolutionary. It was the first, and to my knowledge remains the only, post-graduate practitioner training based entirely within the Wellness & Prevention Paradigm.

Is it lack of evidence that has prevented lifestyle intervention from becoming the foundation of healthcare or a lack of acceptance and implementation of this evidence into clinical mainstream thinking and practice?

I am also very proud to say that all practitioners are welcomed, not only to register, but by all the attendees. The programs are unique and exemplary in creating an environment that puts patient outcomes above professional affiliation. I am also grateful to Parker Seminars for providing me a platform to educate practitioners; without them I would not have been able to introduce my ideas and concepts to the profession. Having the opportunity to lecture to thousands of practitioners at Parker Seminars has been instrumental to accomplishing my mission to catalyze the Wellness & Prevention Paradigm movement. I am pleased to publicly acknowledge and thank both Dr. Mancini and Dr. Lamarche, presidents of Parker College and Parker Seminars, respectively.

I am also extremely proud of the practitioners who attend the programs and the lectures I present. These practitioners, mostly chiropractors at this juncture, do not have a pharmaceutical company paying their seminar fees or their travel expenses or for their missed time in practice. These practitioners pay their own way for the sole purpose of learning ways to improve the health outcomes of their patients. They don't charge more money for these improved patient outcomes, most of them provide free lifestyle workshops for their patients. Many of these chiropractors have also paid me to come and speak to their communities and have invited other practitioners including general practitioners, orthopedic surgeons, hospital administrators, naturopaths, homeopaths, physiotherapists, massage therapists, and, in fact, anyone else who wishes to attend. Being focused on finding the best evidence to help people get and stay well just naturally brings together those who put patient interests first.

I have spoken in large theaters, in large churches, at universities and colleges and in large community centers all over the world and the spirit is always about working together, practitioners and patients, to create longer, better lives. There is hope and there is good reason for optimism.

Does your practitioner provide wellness and prevention workshops?

I often get asked two questions. The first is why I chose to become a chiropractor instead of a medical doctor. Actually my real decision was between accepting a fellowship to do a Ph.D. and chiropractic college because by the time I made this decision, which was after I completed my Master of Science degree in exercise physiology, I had already decided that what I wanted to do with my life was prevent illness and promote health rather than diagnose and treat disease.

To be honest I was strongly leaning toward completing the Ph.D. My father is a Ph.D. biologist and I had strong influences to pursue this path (family history, must be genetic). I wanted to look at preventing osteoporosis, falls, and hip fractures in the elderly with exercise and balance training. I was very ambitious. I had already been reading a great deal about wellness and prevention. I had just read the book 'Perfect Health' by Deepak Chopra and I was really very enthusiastic about creating a different type of care.

I had done quite a bit of research on aging and the positive benefits of exercise in the elderly. I had a lot of statistics on the costs associated with the PREVENTABLE issues of osteoporosis, falls, and hip fractures, and the great number of early deaths, and great loss of quality of life, associated with these issues. I really was ready to change the world. I had already envisioned and planned out the revolutionary facility I was going to operate and how much money I would save the system and how many lives I would improve and prolong. I was so focused and so sure about my plan that I contacted the Medical Services Plan in British Columbia because I wanted to find out about what kind of funding I would be able to get after I finished my Ph.D. and had become a world leading expert in preventing osteoporosis, falls, and hip fractures in the elderly.

The answer shocked me. The answer was NONE. The Medical Services Plan, the socialized, tax-payer funded healthcare system, did not pay for any care that was not provided by a medical doctor. The criteria for paying for a service had nothing to do with evidence, nothing to do with ability to prove expertise, it was based solely on whether or not you were an "approved" practitioner. The medical profession had a monopoly regarding government funding for healthcare interventions and I was told with certainty that, regardless of how much evidence I had, that this was not going to change. At the time I had no concept of charging people directly for a health service, it was just outside my paradigm. I said to the woman I was speaking to, "do you mean that if I actually conduct the research that provides unequivocal evidence that my exercise and nutrition and mind-body/relaxation/stress reduction program prevents osteoporosis, prevents falls, saves lives and saves millions of dollars that you won't pay for that service." She confirmed I was correct. I asked if there was any other such program in place. She confirmed there was not. This was the first of many shocking discoveries I have had regarding healthcare.

How is what interventions are funded by government or third party payers determined? Is it based on which interventions have the most evidence, which ones work best, or by which practitioners have a monopoly as insured providers?

I was at a crossroads. I did not want to be a professor, teaching at a university would keep me too far removed from the citizens I wanted to help. I wanted to work directly with patients but I did not want to be a Sickness & Treatment practitioner; I wanted to be a Wellness & Prevention practitioner. I started to look into my options. There were few, in fact as it turns out none. I settled for the closest option available. I had already had an incredibly positive experience with chiropractic. After a very serious rugby injury, and a very long and painful year without relief within the medical system, and against the advice of my medical doctor who told me chiropractic was dangerous, out of desperation I went to a chiropractor and got incredible, life changing results. Ironically when I told my medical doctor this he was anything but thrilled. He showed absolutely no joy for the fact that I was finally recovering.

He was more interested in who helped me than whether or not I got helped. That really affected me and to this day I am determined to help create a system that is focused on helping patients not on which practitioner gets credit.

I just can't tell you how repugnant it is to me to allow arrogance and ignorance to get in the way of patient care. To me that is criminal negligence, it is malpractice, it is a flagrant violation of the Hippocratic Oath.

When I looked into chiropractic something very important jumped out at me. The mission statement of chiropractic was that treating symptoms alone was not logical and that the focus of healthcare professionals should be finding and addressing the cause of illness and removing interferences from the natural, innate self healing and self regulating abilities of the person with the illness. This, by far, represented the closest thing I could find to a wellness and prevention healthcare field.

What is more important, if someone gets well or which practitioner provided the intervention?

Now I would like to point out two very important things. One, chiropractic care alone is not capable of addressing all the causes of illness or supplying all the things required to restore the innate self healing and self regulating abilities; that would be a dangerously illogical stance. Chiropractic alone is not a treatment solution for chronic illness, it is, however, a vitally important intervention, and in fact the most evidence-based intervention, if you have a lack of motion in your spinal or extremity joints.

Chiropractic certainly can remove rocks out of the backpack, allostatic loads, that are associated with lack of motion in the spinal and extremity joints and tissues. The research is clear that a lack of proper motion in synovial joints represents a stressor, an allostatic load, and that proper motion and alignment of joints is a genetic requirement for the expression of physical and mental health.[105] We need healthy spines. Healthy spines move well and send healthy afferent neurological signals (proprioception) to the brain. These signals are important for brain function and, via neurological and neurobiochemical pathways, for brain controlled function of the entire human ecosystem and human experience.[106]

Chiropractic is important for health for many of the same reasons exercise is so important for overall health. Movement feeds the brain, the movement nutrients are afferent nerve signals called proprioception that travel from properly moving joints to the brain. There are well documented movement-learning and movement-pleasure pathways that involve the spinal joints and surrounding tissues sending proprioceptive signals to the brain.[107, 108, 109] Proper range of motion is required for this to occur. Chiropractic can help restore motion and thus the delivery of motion-derived nutrients (proprioception) to the brain. Of course you still need to exercise. Chiropractic can help restore range of motion, it cannot provide sufficient motion.

Can a human being be healthy without a healthy, properly moving and aligned spine?

When your spinal joints are not moving properly they start to degenerate and get inflamed and they send stress signals (nociception) to the brain that can lead to the brain releasing the stress hormones involved in chronic stress physiology (cortisol and catecholamines). This can also, but does not always, lead to pain.[110] Restoring motion decreases these stress signals, decreases the stress hormone release they elicit, and thus decreases allostatic load. If the nociception is caused solely by the lack of motion and proprioception, pain will almost certainly subside when motion and proprioception are restored and nociception is reduced. However, if there are other sources of nociception, if there are other unaddressed rocks in the backpack, the pain may not subside. The restoration of motion is required, and beneficial, whether the pain subsides or not. Remember the plant analogy? The plant can still be wilting even after receiving water and improving function – it may also need nutrients or sunlight or the removal of toxins. The same is true for back pain or any other symptom.

There are very few health issues that are caused by one stressor or rock in the backpack and even fewer that are solved by the removal of one stressor or rock in the backpack. This is precisely why a holistic approach that includes lifestyle is so important.

Whether this improvement in spinal motion and the restoration of the afferent neurological pathways involved with restored proprioception and reduced nociception can treat or cure any chronic disease is not the relevant or important question if the goal is improving health and function. The only things that are relevant are whether or not a lack of proper motion is a stress load and detracts from health and whether or not restoring this motion removes that stress load and improves or restores the health and function that was lost due to the lack of motion. The science is clear, lack of motion degenerates joints and causes decreased proprioception and increased nociception.[111, 112] The science is also clear that these changes can lead to significant increases in stress load and stress hormone release. There is also peer-reviewed research to show that chiropractic spinal adjustments result in restored motion (proprioception) and reduced nociception and stress hormone levels.[113, 114, 115, 116,117]

In terms of the cause of chronic illness and the requirements for chronic health is it logical to assume a single cause or single solution?

Now, if anyone ever tries to tell you that there is no evidence to support chiropractic they are either deliberately lying, simply ignorant of the literature, or expressing a falsehood which is based on either misinformation or dogmatic bias. Again, let me be very clear. This does not mean chiropractic is a valid or logical treatment for chronic illness. Does this mean that patients under chiropractic care never see improvements in chronic illness symptom or risk factor status? Certainly not. There are a great many chiropractic patients with documented improvements in things like immune function, asthma, allergies, colic, blood pressure, cholesterol levels, depression, anxiety and many other things. The same is true for people who have received any intervention that reduces stress load or allostatic load. The same is true for people who start to exercise (or remove the stress of sedentary living), for people who reduce emotional stress with meditation and imagery, for people who improve their diets etc.

Any intervention that removes toxicity and/or deficiency and/ or restores purity and sufficiency moves us toward health and away from adaptive physiology. Whether such interventions alone will "cure" a disease is not what determines their worth. What determines their worth is whether or not they reduce allostatic load and improve states of health and function.

Without doubt, there will certainly always be other stressors or allostatic loads or rocks in the backpack that need to be addressed. Suggesting there is one cause (bad genes) and one cure or treatment (drugs) for chronic illness is just not a logical or scientifically sound approach.

How is an improvement in overall health status possible from improving spinal motion? It is not magic. Reducing a stress load, removing a rock from the backpack, reduces the release of stress hormones and pushes you up the scale of health and function away from stress physiology and toward homeostatic physiology. This can, but does not always, result in a change in seemingly unrelated (but actually very related) physiology and symptoms.

Let me help you understand. There is a lot of misinformation and confusion about chiropractic, some of it deliberately spread, some just a product of a lack of understanding by both chiropractors and other health professionals. Once you understand the effects of elevated stress hormones you can begin to understand that anything that elevates them represents a stress load or allostatic load or rock in the backpack. Understanding this requires viewing things through the Wellness & Prevention Paradigm. The question must change from whether a lack of spinal motion is the singular cause of any specific symptom or chronic disease to whether or not lack of spinal motion represents a stress load and thus a contributing causal factor in loss of function and health.

If an intervention removes a stressor from your internal or external environment, does this intervention, by definition, result in greater health and function?

The question must change from whether chiropractic care alone represents a treatment for symptoms or chronic disease to whether restoring joint motion represents a removal or reduction of stress load (allostatic load) and thus a move toward better health and function.

Let me share with you what can be substantiated with valid scientific evidence. Lack of proper spinal motion causes spinal joints to degenerate and become inflamed and this causes an increase in body stress signals (nociception) to be sent to the brain. Increased nociceptive signals cause the brain to increase the release of stress hormones such as cortisol and catecholamines. Increased release of stress hormones drives the physiology of the body toward a state of alarm and adaptation, and, if these levels remain elevated, fatigue, illness, and early death (a summary of the effects of these hormones was provided in an earlier chapter).

I have not said that a lack of spinal motion by itself can cause a large enough increase in stress hormones to cause chronic illness or early death; there is no evidence to either substantiate or deny this. I have said that a lack of spinal motion can cause an increase in these stress hormones that contribute (along with all the other stressors or rocks in the backpack) to the expression of adaptive physiology. Lack of spinal motion represents an allostatic load and thus, without question, you are healthier with proper motion than you are without, regardless of what disease or symptoms you have or don't have. Sometimes removing this allostatic load results in significant changes in clinical signs and symptoms and sometimes it just results in better health and function without a change in symptoms.

To suggest that the millions of patients who have reported significant health improvements under chiropractic care are lying or simply experienced a 'placebo effect' is scientifically absurd.

If lack of proper spinal motion represents a stressor, if it represents an allostatic load, if it results in adaptive physiology, does it represent a causal factor in chronic illness?

First of all these patients almost always report that they were not expecting these results at all, that they, and often the chiropractor, were completely surprised that they occurred. Second, many chiropractic patients have anything but a blind faith in chiropractic when they begin care. It is usually, and regrettably, a last resort.

Again, please understand. None of these facts make it ethical, logical, or scientific to claim chiropractic alone is a valid treatment for chronic disease. What these facts do ethically, logically, and scientifically suggest is that every person, regardless of disease, is better off with a healthy moving spine than without one and that chiropractic is an ethical, logical and evidence-based intervention to restore motion in joints and surrounding tisues. Isn't the same true for having a healthy attitude or utilizing stress reduction? Do we know exactly what disease you will get if you are angry and resentful and stressed out? No we don't. Do we have enough evidence to suggest that being angry and resentful and stressed out is unhealthy? Yes we do. Does this mean that meditation and positive thinking alone is a valid treatment for disease? No it does not. Does it mean that, regardless of diagnosis, people will benefit from moving away from anger and resentment and emotional stress and toward a state of relaxation and forgiveness? Yes it does. It is all about the paradigm. It is about the questions we ask. Again, remember the plant analogy.

By the way a lack of proper motion in your spinal joints also results in a decrease in proprioceptive messages being sent to your brain, particularly the cerebellum and the cerebellar-hippocampal and cerebellar-hypothalamic pathways involved in the movement-learning and movement-pleasure pathways. There is just so much information to support the idea that, regardless of disease or symptoms, humans are much healthier with a properly moving spine than without. For the life of me I cannot understand how this can be controversial or confusing. It certainly is not due to a lack of science; it can only be due to a lack of understanding of, or willingness to accept, the science.

The areas of reduced or restricted spinal motion causing the spinal degeneration and the changes in neurological communication between body and brain are termed vertebral subluxation complex.[118] Think of them as cavities. They can be present without pain or with pain.Getting rid of them requires a doctor who has training and expertise in detecting and correcting them. Preventing them requires brushing and flossing (spinal range of motion and postural exercises). They are common.

Is sitting for hours each day and living a sedentary industrial life as hard on the spine as sugar is to our teeth?

Sitting to your spine is like sugar to your teeth. Subluxation complex is common within industrial society because we have a pandemic of sedentary living, because we have traumas from accidents and sports, because few if any move their spinal joints through the full range of motion on a regular basis, and because we now sit for most of our lives.

Our industrial lifestyle is as genetically incompatible for our spines as it is for our teeth and for every other aspect of our health. If you have a spine and you live in industrial society you will benefit from having a chiropractor check your spine for subluxation complex just like you benefit from having a dentist check your teeth for cavities. If your spinal joints are not moving properly a chiropractor needs to get them moving properly and to give you proper spinal hygiene exercises and other lifestyle advice so YOU can do your best to keep them moving. I promise it really is not complicated or mysterious or illogical or unscientific. The improvements in health you get will be consistent. The improvements in symptoms or illness status will depend on how many other rocks you have in your backpack.

There it is, chiropractic in a nutshell. Spinal joints not moving properly represent rocks in your backpack. Restoring motion to spinal joints represents removing rocks from your backpack. It is that simple. No magic, no hocus pocus, no magic and no miracles. Just expected results based on spinal joint motion, the associated afferent body – brain neurological and neurobiochemical communication pathways, and changes in the efferent brain - body neurological and neurobiochemical regulation of global physiology.

Anyone who suggests to you that it is not important to ensure you have a healthy moving spine is quite simply dangerously ignorant or deliberately dishonest. Any chiropractor who tells you that restoring motion to your spine alone is a valid treatment for chronic disease is either dangerously ignorant, highly unethical, or both. Any chiropractor who explains that a healthy moving spine is necessary for healthy spinal joints and tissues and also for healthy body-brain neurological communication which is important for overall health is a practitioner you want to add to your healthcare team. If they also offer a lifestyle program that teaches you about the importance of lifestyle, which lifestyle choices are genetically congruent, how to implement and sustain these choices, and that measures and records your progress and health outcomes, then they should be the LEADER of your healthcare team. I would say the same about any practitioner who offers such a program. I can't emphasize this enough, it is not the profession that matters, it is the interventions and the health outcomes they elicit that determine the value of practitioner and intervention.

If joint motion produces essential nutrient stimulation for our brains called proprioception, are we deficient in this nutrient if our joints cannot move through their full range of motion?

This brings me to the next important thing to point out. Many chiropractic colleges and chiropractors are now operating completely within the Sickness & Treatment Paradigm; they have moved away from the original tenets of chiropractic and moved toward focusing solely on the treatment of back pain and other physical symptoms rather than on restoring health and function. The reasons for this are numerous and complicated but this discussion is not appropriate here. Needless to say much of this has had to do with trying to get accepted into, or trying to prevent being attacked by, the Sickness & Treatment Paradigm system. You will get more insight into this in the next chapter.

What is appropriate here is for me to be ethical and to meet my moral obligation to tell you that simply because someone is a chiropractor does not mean that they are offering care that is within the Wellness & Prevention Paradigm. I am NOT an advocate for any profession, I am an advocate for patients. My loyalty is to patients and to patient outcomes. Again, it is not the initials after the name that determines patient outcomes, it is the ability of the intervention to elicit improved health outcomes. This is all that matters to me and it is all that should matter to you.

There are some progressive chiropractic colleges that are trying to incorporate the content of the post-graduate wellness lifestyle program into the curriculum but this is difficult because it would have to replace an existing part of their curriculum or add more courses to an already overwhelming work load.

What healthcare profession has the Wellness & Prevention Paradigm foundational concepts that the body is intelligent, self healing and regulating, and that addressing the cause of illness is of paramount importance?

I think the future will see wellness and prevention being a specialty choice at chiropractic colleges and probably at other healthcare professional schools.

The reasons I have felt it is more pragmatic to approach and work with the chiropractic profession before other professions are twofold. One, chiropractors have always had the concepts of the body being intelligent, self healing, and self regulating and addressing the cause of illness as the foundation of their education and practice. Yes this may have come to be focused on addressing the cause of spinal pain and other symptoms among some elements of the profession but the basic concept of addressing the cause and the fact that the body is innately intelligent and self healing and regulating are still deeply engrained. Obviously a profession that has the major foundational premise that the body is genetically strong rather than weak and that cell function is naturally healthy not pathologically sick is going to more readily embrace the Wellness & Prevention Paradigm.

Two, chiropractic operates, or has been forced to operate, largely outside of the established Sickness & Treatment Paradigm system. Chiropractic is free of the inherent bias against 'drugless" practitioners and 'drug-free' interventions and also free of the virtually inextricable relationship with pharmaceutical companies that will undoubtedly be a major obstacle to a change away from a drug centered, sickness and treatment centered system. Personally I hope all professions get involved, I hope that wellness and prevention becomes defined solely by the wellness and prevention knowledge and training of the practitioner and the interventions offered.

I am willing and eager to work with anybody and everybody. We have a real opportunity to get things right in the interest of the patients. However, the most important thing to realize is that delaying implementation costs lives. The choice of which practitioners take this on (hopefully a mix of all healthcare professions) cannot be determined by anything other than who is qualified and ready to do so.

The need and demand for lifestyle practitioners far outweighs the number available and this will remain the case for years to come. We simply have to do whatever is necessary to create as many qualified lifestyle practitioners as quickly as possible. Lives depend on it, about this there is no debate.

When drug-free lifestyle intervention becomes the foundation of healthcare what will be considered "alternative" and what will be considered "mainstream"?.

It may just be, as ironic as this seems, that chiropractic and other drug-free healthcare professions are, for the first time in history, going to have their drug-free status become a great advantage. What are now viewed as 'alternative' or 'complimentary' practitioners within the Sickness & Treatment Paradigm are destined to become the establishment practitioners within the Wellness & Prevention Paradigm. The Wellness & Prevention Paradigm that will inevitably come to dominate healthcare, by economic necessity if not by an acceptance of the evidence, will make the foundation of healthcare practice drug-free; the foundation of 21st century healthcare will by necessity become lifestyle intervention.

Chapter 11 New Paradigm – New Practitioners: Will the Reform Meet Resistance?

The medical monopoly or medical trust is not merely the meanest monopoly ever organized, but the most arrogant, dangerous and despotic ... Any and all methods of healing the sick by means of safe, simple and natural remedies are assailed and denounced as fakes and frauds.

J.W. Hodge M.D.

The hard truth is that once we accept the fact that lifestyle intervention is the most evidence-based, most effective, and most cost-effective solution regarding wellness and prevention, this immediately makes the vast majority of drug and surgical procedures, and any 'natural treatments for disease, and the practitioners that offer them, ineffective at best and harmful at worst. This is a tough pill (or natural herb) to swallow.

Too bad, I could care less about how hard it is or whose feelings might get hurt or whose ego might get bruised or who might lose money or power or influence or social status.

People are dying by the millions, our children are overweight and sick, our elderly are infirm and our middle aged are so sick that 80 percent of our workforce is riddled with chronic illness. Nothing else matters. The only thing that matters is getting and keeping people well.

What letters we have after our name, what schools we went to, what profession we belong to are all MEANINGLESS when it comes to saving lives. The only thing that matters is whether or not what we offer is effective in getting and keeping people well. We need to stop assessing treatments by whether they can change a disease risk factor or a symptom and start assessing interventions by whether or not they can restore health or prevent illness. This is 21st Century healthcare. It's not a matter of if, it is a matter of how long, how many more lives and how many more dollars will be wasted, before when.

There will probably be turf wars. Medical associations and the pharmaceutical companies spent years and billions of dollars lobbying to take control of healthcare.

Their strategy was to pass the drugless practitioner act which divided all practitioners into two categories; those with the legal right to prescribe drugs and perform surgery and 'the rest'. They spent billions of dollars on marketing and lobbying to make everyone believe that only those practitioners that could prescribe drugs were 'real doctors' and scientific and that everyone else was an unscientific 'quack'. Ask yourself what your opinion of non-medical practitioners is. Ask yourself what your medical doctor's opinion of non-medical practitioners is. Are these opinions based on facts, on evidence, on research, or on a long-standing deliberate campaign to create this dogmatic belief system?

What is your opinion of non-medical practitioners? Is this opinion based on evidence or dogma? Is it based on opinions of medical practitioners or on evidence?

Let me give you a quick history lesson. Despite organized medicine's efforts to create a strong bias against non-medical practitioners, a growing number of dissatisified patients began seeking out such practitioners. To combat this loss of power and revenue organized medicine and the pharmaceutical companies who depended on them, and ultimately came to strongly influence them, simply increased their efforts - often illegally.

In 1963 the AMA authorized the formation of the Committee on Quackery whose primary goal was to "contain and eliminate chiropractic." The committee conducted nationwide conferences on chiropractic, prepared and distributed anti-chiropractic propaganda calling chiropractic an unscientific cult, regularly communicated with medical boards and associations warning that professional association between medical physicians and chiropractors was unethical, and actively discouraged colleges, universities, and faculty members from cooperating with chiropractic schools and/or research efforts.[119]

Keeping chiropractors out of hospitals was one of the primary goals of the AMA. When, based on evidence of effectiveness and safety, chiropractic was included under medicare in 1973, the AMA became especially concerned that this would open the way for chiropractors into hospitals. The AMA actually threatened hospitals with loss of accreditation if they allowed chiropractors to come into the hospitals and help patients.[120]

Did you know that in 1987 a Federal U.S. appellate court found the American Medical Association guilty of an illegal, deliberate, disinformation campaign and an organized conspiracy to destroy chiropractic that was based on eliminating competition? Did you know that the AMA repeatedly tried to appeal this decision and that the decision was upheld in the U.S. Court of Appeals in 1990 and that the AMA petitioned the U.S. Supreme Court three separate times for an appeal and each time were denied? Did you know that the judge ordered an injunction that included orders that the AMA cease and desist its efforts to restrict the professional association of chiropractors and AMA members and further, to personally notify all 275,000 of its members of this injunction? Did you know that the American Hospital Association sent out 440,000 separate notices to inform hospitals across the United States that they had no objection to allowing chiropractic care in hospitals? Did you know that during the trial it was conclusively shown that the AMA deliberately and willfully undermined chiropractic education and schools, undercut insurance programs for chiropractic patients, and concealed evidence of the effectiveness of chiropractic care?[121] Did you know that by the time this occurred that the AMA's efforts to undermine the reputation of chiropractic within the medical and public domains had been so successful that this bias still exists and still adversely affects many doctors and patients?

Have the attacks on non-medical practitioners been motivated by evidence of ineffectiveness or harm, by evidence of superiority of medical interventions, or by protection of a monopoly?

Let me give you another history lesson. In 1993 the Ministry of Health in Ontario, Canada commissioned an independent report on the effectiveness and cost-effectiveness of chiropractic management of low back pain. This was an independent report; none of the authors were chiropractors. The head researcher Pran Manga, Ph.D., Professor and Director, Masters in Health Administration Program, University of Ottawa and his co-authors did an exhaustive review of the available literature.[122]

Let me quote directly from this commissioned report regarding the published findings.

"On the evidence, particularly the most scientifically valid clinical studies, spinal manipulation applied by chiropractors is shown to be more effective than alternative treatments for low back pain. Many medical therapies are of questionable validity or are clearly inadequate." "Our reading of the literature suggests that chiropractic manipulation is safer than medical management of low back pain." "What the literature revealed to us is the much greater need for clinical evidence of the validity of medical management of low back pain."[123]

"Indeed, several existing medical therapies for low back pain are generally contraindicated on the basis of existing trials. There is also some evidence in the literature to suggest that spinal manipulations are less safe and less effective when performed by non-chiropractic professionals." "There is an overwhelming body of evidence indicating that chiropractic management of low-back pain is more cost-effective than medical management. The lack of any convincing argument or evidence to the contrary must be noted and is significant to us in forming our conclusions and recommendations. The evidence includes studies showing lower chiropractic costs for the same diagnosis and episodic need for care."

What is your opinion of chiropractic? Is it possible you have the opinion that it is either unscientific or unsafe? Where did this opinion come from? Is it from reading the literature or from dogmatic opinion?

"There would be highly significant cost savings if more management of low back pain was transferred from physicians to chiropractors. Evidence from Canada and other countries suggests potential savings of hundreds of millions annually."[124]

"Despite official medical disapproval and economic disincentive to patients (higher private out-of-pocket cost), the use of chiropractic has grown steadily over the years."

"In our view, the constellation of the evidence of:

1. The effectiveness and cost-effectiveness of chiropractic management of low back pain

2. The untested, questionable or harmful nature of many current medical therapies

3. The economic efficiency of chiropractic care for low back pain compared with medical care

4. The safety of chiropractic care

5. The higher satisfaction levels expressed by patients of chiropractors. Together this evidence offers an overwhelming case in favour of much greater use of chiropractic services in the management of low back pain."

Based on these findings, the recommendations of the Manga Report were as follows:

1. "There should be a shift in policy to encourage and prefer chiropractic services for most patients with low back pain."

If you compared and contrasted the EVIDENCE regarding safety, cost-effectiveness, effectiveness, and patient satisfaction for all available spinal care interventions which would be valuated the highest?

2. "Chiropractic services should be fully insured under the Ontario Health Insurance Plan, removing the economic disincentive for patients and referring health providers."

3. "Because of the high incidence and cost of low back pain, hospitals, managed health care groups (community health centers, comprehensive health organizations, and health service organizations) and long-term care facilities should employ chiropractors on a full-time and/or part-time basis."

4. "Chiropractors should be employed by tertiary hospitals in Ontario. The opportunity for consultation, second opinion and wider treatment options are significant advantages we foresee from this initiative which has been employed with success in a clinical research setting at the University Hospital, Saskatoon."

5. "Hospital privileges should be extended to all chiropractors for the purposes of treatment of their own patients who have been hospitalized for other reasons, and for access to diagnostic facilities relevant to their scope of practice and patients' needs."

6. "Chiropractors should have access to all pertinent patient records and tests from hospitals, physicians, and other health care professionals upon the consent of their patients. Access should be given upon the request of chiropractors or their patients."

7. "Since low back pain is of such significant concern to workers' compensation, chiropractors should be engaged at a senior level by Workers' Compensation Board to assess policy, procedures, and treatment of workers with back injuries." "A very good case can be made for making chiropractors the gatekeepers for management of low back pain in the workers' compensation system in Ontario."

8. "Chiropractic education in Ontario should be in the multidisciplinary atmosphere of a university with appropriate funding. Chiropractic is the only regulated health profession in Ontario without public funding for education at present, and it works against the best interests of the health care system for chiropractors to be educated in relative isolation from other health science students."

9. "Finally, the government should take all reasonable steps to actively encourage cooperation between providers, particularly the chiropractic, medical, and physiotherapy professions. Lack of cooperation has been a major factor in the current inefficient management of low back pain."

Why would an independently commissioned report, whose recommendations could save billions of dollars, be ignored?

This report was one of the main reasons, other than paradigm, that I chose to enter the chiropractic profession. This report made me realize that my own previous bias, and the bias of so many I discussed my consideration of becoming a chiropractor with, including my own Ph.D. father and some of the Ph.D. professors at the university where I was completing my Master of Science degree, was based on unscientific, dogmatic, unethical opinion and not scientifically valid information. Ironically and most hypocritically, it is often these same people that accuse chiropractic of being unscientific and dogmatic.

Can you guess how many of these recommendations were implemented? None. You can imagine how this report was received by those whose living and social status were, and remain, dependent upon perpetuation of the drug and surgery centered system. The lobbyists from the medical and pharmaceutical industries put more resources into blocking these recommendations than could be competed with.

This is neither evidence that all medical doctors are unethical nor that all chiropractors are. It is just indisputable evidence that the opinions that you, your medical doctor, and your friends and coworkers have about drug-free practitioners have almost certainly been influenced by deliberate dogmatic, biased, unethical propaganda. Most tragically this has resulted in millions of people not being helped who could have been and millions receiving back surgeries and drugs that were ineffective and in many cases caused great harm. For what? For power and money. Healthcare is supposed to be free of this, healthcare deals with people who are so vulnerable and with practitioners whose statements and opinions have so much influence. We owe patients every effort to do better in the 21st century. All unfounded prejudices, whether racial, professional, or otherwise, eventually get exposed as ugly and harmful, as do those who continue to espouse such prejudices. It is difficult to be a minority among any unethical majority, regardless of whether this is based on race, age, gender, wealth, or social status. As Martin Luther King taught us all, it is not whether or not a minority stance is easy or difficult, or popular or unpopular, that should ever determine whether or not we take such a stance.

What is the moral obligation of all health care practitioners? Is it to be loyal to a profession or loyal to the best interests of patients?

This would never happen now though would it? Tragically, yes, it is still happening. As more and more evidence comes to light about the ineffectiveness and dangers of drugs and surgery, and of the relatively or comparatively higher effectiveness and safety of chiropractic, those who have a vested interest in maintaining the medical monopoly at any cost have had to come up with another way to try to undermine competition. The latest false anti-chiropractic propaganda is about the danger of injury or stroke. Although the peer-reviewed evidence clearly shows this propaganda to be false, the damage has already been done and once again millions who could benefit from the greater safety and effectiveness of a drug-free intervention will continue to suffer.

Just a few years ago in Canada a neurologist was found to have deliberately falsified data regarding chiropractic and the risk of stroke. He got this false data and his false conclusions and recommendations published in the Canadian Medical Association Journal and letters were sent to neurologists across Canada warning them about the dangers of chiropractic. [125, 126, 127]

A similar campaign is now going on in Connecticut in the United States where 'awareness groups' have paid to put up anti-chiropractic billboards and signs on buses. Ironically, these people are trying to use the same propaganda that has already been completely discredited in courts in Canada and, more importantly, in the peer-reviewed literature. One can't help but wonder where these people get their funding. One need not wonder at all where they get their motivation.

Why do I include this information? Certainly not to make the case that this suggests that every chiropractor or other drugless practitioner is virtuous or that every medical practitioner is not. Nothing could be further from the truth. I include this so that you will use unbiased scientific evidence and experience rather than biased, dogmatic propaganda to form your opinions and make your decisions. I include it so that you can check yourself and make sure that you form your opinions, and seek your advice, based on what intervention a practitioner offers rather than the profession the practitioner belongs to.

What is most important, what profession a health care practitioner belongs to or what improvements in health outcomes their interventions elicit?

Don't let dogma and prejudice, regarding any practitioner or healthcare profession, get in your way of getting well. There are honest, intelligent, ethical practitioners in every healthcare profession and every healthcare profession has its share of unethical, dishonest individuals.

In fairness and with respect I want to include the fact that many medical practitioners, including general practitioners, neurologists, and surgeons, have come forward and spoken out against bias and for the importance of interdisciplinary efforts to ensure the best care possible for patients and to stop dogmatic prejudice against any practitioner that was 'drugless' or outside the medical profession. Certainly things are changing but change is too slow when it comes to saving lives. We can't afford to wait for professions to change, we need individuals to change NOW.

Let me end this topic with a positive story. A few years ago I was asked by a chiropractic association to come and present to the medical students at a medical school. The medical school was exposing their students to "complementary" healthcare and they had contacted the state chiropractic association to ask if they would like to participate. Although I was not a member of their association, I had recently presented at their annual convention recently and they felt I would be a good "ringer" to bring up to bat (or perhaps sheep to throw to the wolves!).

The medical doctor organizing the event gathered us together before we met the students and told us that we should not be worried about having to provide evidence for what we did but rather that we should simply tell the students that we were there to tell them what we do rather than why we do it. I stated emphatically that I would refuse to participate if I could not discuss evidence. I said that the very thing that was required most in order to change bias was to change the false belief system that chiropractic was less evidence-based than medicine. I said addressing this issue was the only reason I was there. With some resistance he agreed. The first thing I told the students when I got into the classroom was that I was a scientist by training, that I loved evidence-based discussion, that I was very familiar with the literature, and that I was aware of some of the biases they might have. I promised I would not be offended by any question they asked. In fact, I insisted that asking the tough questions was the only way I would get the opportunity to answer them.

How do we know if an opinion is based on dogmatic bias, sound logic, or valid evidence?

Well, with a little hesitation the first hand went up. I thanked the young student for her courage and asked her to ask her question. She said, and I quote, "We just came from anatomy lab and our teacher was showing us the vertebral artery and told us that a chiropractic adjustment or manipulation can cause damage to this artery and cause a stroke, what is your opinion on this?" I said that my opinion was not important, I said the literature and the evidence were important. I asked her if her instructor shared evidence or opinion. She said she wasn't sure. I said, "did your instructor quote any literature to substantiate that chiropractic caused stroke?" She said no. I said "then your instructor shared opinion". I then said that we should now determine if that was accurate, evidence-based opinion or another classification of opinion.

I asked the student if she had ever seen any evidence that chiropractic caused stroke. She said no but that she had heard something about it. I asked her if she was familiar with any of the peer-reviewed evidence on the issue. She said no. I then asked her colleagues the same question. None of them were. I then asked them if they would like to be. They said yes. I thanked them for being so professional and scientific and then I handed them all a copy of a paper I had recently published on the issue of chiropractic and stroke entitled 'The Stroke Issue: Paucity of Valid Data, Plethora of Unsubstantiated Conjecture."[128]

I asked them if they were familiar with the fact that the literature studying the stresses put on the vertebral artery during a chiropractic adjustment were, in the words of the researcher, Walter Herzog, PhD from the Biomechanics Department at the University of Calgary, less than what occurs during normal active and passive range of motion.[129] In other words, a chiropractic adjustment or manipulation results in less strain on the vertebral artery than turning your head. They were not aware of this either.

In the end we all agreed that, as doctors, our moral obligation was to form our opinions based on science and evidence and to demand that those providing opinions should do the same.

This was the only way we could put the interest of the patients, rather than any profession or practitioner, first, and it was certainly what the Hippocratic Oath, which I had already taken, and they would soon take, was designed to accomplish. Once these students realized I formed my opinions based on evidence, and once they realized that their pre-formed opinions about chiropractic were not formed on evidence, they changed from skeptics into soon to be doctors trying to become familiar with the evidence regarding if and when chiropractic might help their future patients. It was, and remains, one of the most positive and optimistic experiences of my lecturing career.

What is the intent of the Hippocratic Oath?

At the end we were all just doctors, with different skill sets and knowledge bases, working toward the common goal of helping patients. It was exactly what healthcare should be. It was dogma and bias-free discussion of evidence with the single-minded goal of serving patients – it was a brief utopia!

You are the consumer, you are responsible to choose which type of intervention best meets your needs. Make this choice based on evidence and knowledge not dogma and prejudice. Most importantly understand that any type of practitioner can be entrenched in the Sickness & Treatment Paradigm and any type of practitioner can be entrenched in the Wellness & Prevention Paradigm. It is the paradigm that determines what kind of intervention will be offered not the profession.

The irony of the drugless practitioner act and all the bias it has caused is that when it comes to wellness and prevention nothing could be less evidence-based, less effective, or more 'quacky' than drugs and surgery.

Regardless of the past the most important point is that the future, 21st century healthcare, must not be about one paradigm OR the other but rather one paradigm AND the other. It must not be about one profession or practitioner OR the other but rather ALL professions and practitioners working together, in an evidence-based way, to provide the best care possible for the patient.

The Hippocratic Oath is not an oath of allegiance to any particular profession, it is an oath of allegiance to patients. It's time we all put the patient first.

What is the difference between science and dogma?

Science is based on the encouragement of logic and independent thinking, questioning, and critique. Dogma is based on the encouragement of blind faith and acceptance of concepts or ideas or strategies put forward by accepted leaders. Your health and the health of your loved ones are too important to allow dogma to guide your decisions.

Moral, ethical healthcare systems and providers are scientific, not dogmatic. As soon as you hear someone tell you that they know everything and that nobody else knows anything, run. None of us know enough.

I have put a great body of evidence together for you, and I'm very confident that what I'm sharing with you is correct, but as soon as I stop wanting to learn, or think that if someone thinks differently than me, or isn't a member of my social network or peer group, or doesn't have the same initials after their name, that they must be wrong, I become dogmatic rather than scientific; I become dangerous. Dogma plus power and influence is is not just dangerous, it has proven to be deadly.

Chapter 12
Creating a Working Model: The Innate Lifestyle™ Program

"Things may come to those who wait, but only things left by those who hustle."

Abraham Lincoln

In the end I think a big part of creating the paradigm shift will be having a working model that provides incontrovertible evidence that lifestyle intervention is a pragmatic approach in daily clinical practice. As more and more evidence is published the debate can no longer be about whether or not lifestyle is the cause of chronic illness or that lifestyle change is the only logical solution. The only debate moving forward is whether or not patients will actually make such changes. This is the mantra of the drug companies, drug prescribing physicians, and surgeons who choose to do everything possible to resist change. They make ridiculous statements about patients being unwilling to change and claim that because of this continuing to prescribe drugs to palliate the symptoms of lifestyle caused chronic illness or continuing to perform heart bypass or gastric bypass surgeries are the only real practical clinical approaches.

This is ABSURD. First of all, they make these statements based on the fact that their patients, few if any of whom have ever been educated about the importance of lifestyle, few if any of whom have ever been empowered with the knowledge and skills regarding how to change, few if any of whom have ever been offered a program to help them change, and most if not all of whom have been prescribed medication, seem unwilling to change their lifestyle habits. Are you kidding me? Why would we ever consider that physicians with no training in wellness and prevention, little to no knowledge of the relationships between lifestyle and illness or lifestyle and wellness and prevention, no skill set or programs to offer to empower patients to change, no compensation for spending time on lifestyle, and a belief system that wellness and prevention is useless or impossible, are good judges of whether or not lifestyle intervention is clinically practical? No more.

No more allowing experts in sickness and treatment to offer uneducated, biased opinions about wellness and prevention. This just has to stop, it is costing lives.

I, along with my team of two other doctors and a full-time computer programmer, have spent the last three years developing a working lifestyle intervention model. We have created the Eat Well – Move Well – Think Well™ Innate Lifestyle™ Program for clinicians to educate, inspire, coach, and empower patients regarding healthy lifestyle change. The program is a 12 month applied education program that includes monthly workshops on eating well, moving well, and thinking (and interacting) well. The program includes measurements and ratings of health and vitality, lifestyle allostatic load, and lifestyle wellness and prevention. There are biometric, physical function, and questionnaire data gathered from, and reported to, every participant at 0, 3, 6, 9, and 12 months. The participants each have on-line success journals where they both record, and receive positive feedback for, implementation of the lifestyle behaviors assigned at the workshops. We record all the data and we monitor participation for both the success journal and the workshops via email messages to both participants and practitioners.

Are the wellness and prevention benefits associated with healthy lifestyle change seen if the lifestyle behavior changes are not sustained?

This program is revolutionary for several reasons. First, it is a 12 month program that records actual lifestyle behavior change. The truth is that all the data on preventing chronic illness and saving money with lifestyle programs is only valid if the lifestyle changes are sustained. Putting patients through a short program of a few months and reporting the risk factor, physical function, or biometric improvements is misleading.

If the lifestyle behavior changes are not sustained these improvements are not translated into actual reductions in chronic illness, actual prevention of chronic illness, or actual cost savings. In fact, if you spend money on a lifestyle or wellness program that does not result in long term sustained change you have actually increased costs.

All you have done is spent money to get a short term improvement that has no long term effect. You have just added the cost of an ineffective wellness and prevention program to the costs of drugs and surgery. We created a program to elicit, measure, and track sustained lifestyle behavior change.

What is more likely to be sustained, easy, comfortable, gradual change, or difficult, uncomfortable, sudden change?

This also allows the program to be gradual. If you want change to be sustained it has to meet some very strict criteria. The change has to be meaningful to the person; this means you have to educate about why we get sick, how to get and stay well, and what choices represent genetically congruent eating, moving, and thinking. The change has to be easy, gradual, and comfortable; this means you have to implement easy, gradual, comfortable lifestyle changes that build confidence and momentum with repetition and practice (build healthy habits). The change has to be shown to increase desired outcomes and decrease undesired outcomes; this means that daily, positive feedback regarding the attainment of personal goals has to be included. If you want the program to be clinically practical it has to be easily delivered in a clinical setting. It has to be affordable for participants, represent an excellent return on investment for employers or insurance companies, and be ethically and fairly profitable for the practitioner. We have designed the Innate Lifestyle™ Program to meet all of these criteria.

We just launched the program last year and we now have over 40 centers.

We have centers in the United States, in Canada, in the United Kingdom, and in Australia. I am excited to announce that Life University in Atlanta has just chosen to include the Innate Lifestyle™ Program as an option for their chiropractic interns in their outpatient teaching clinic.

This represents the first practitioners in any healthcare field in history to graduate with the knowledge, skills, and working program to offer evidence-based lifestyle intervention. Dr. Guy Riekeman, the president of Life University, is a visionary. He is also working very hard to include the content of my wellness lifestyle program into the undergraduate curriculum of the university and as part of the chiropractic college curriculum. Lives will be saved because of his efforts and, as always, when he creates a successful model others will quickly follow. Thank you Dr. Riekeman and Life University.

Our ultimate goal is to have the Innate Lifestyle™ Program part of every elementary and high school curriculum. Learning how to eat, move, think, and interact in healthy ways is the most important thing we can teach our children.

The program will represent a revolutionary teaching tool for educators and a phenomenal learning experience for students. We are determined to make the world a healthier place.

We, and our founding licensed Innate Lifestyle™ Program centers, are very excited about what The Innate Lifestyle™ Program is already accomplishing. The Innate Lifestyle™ Program elicits sustainable behavior change and, because our participants access and fill out their success journals on a daily basis, we have the data. As of December 22, 2010 we have had 87,346 success journal days completed. Keep in mind that the bulk of our participants are still in the early months of the program, and thus still in the early phases of their easy, gradual, and comfortable healthy behavior addition. Even so, this number is the equivalent of 239 person-years of data collection. I am not aware of any other lifestyle program that offers such valuable data regarding behavior patterns to patients, practitioners, employers, and payees.

In terms of actual behavioral change, our participants have logged a total of 237,601,219 steps for a total distance of 101,870 miles (163,945 kilometers). That's the equivalent of 4 times around the earth at the equator and it's also an average of 1.2 miles per person per day. Remember, as many of our participants are early in their program, they are only just beginning to add movement into their lives. Our participants have also performed a collective total of 514,850 pushups, 882,835 standing squats and 1,761,076 minutes of aerobic activity (an average of 20 minutes per day).

Summary:

Total steps logged:	237,601,219
Total distance (mi/km):	101,870/163,945
Average distance/person/day (mi/km):	1.2/1.9

Our participants have consumed a total of 520,568 cups of water (an average of 6 cups per person per day); and 456,782 servings of fruits and vegetables (an average of 5.2). As health is the genetic expression of our lifestyle behaviors we are not surprised to see the concomitant improvements in the indices of health we measure during the regular progress assessments. Our participants are seeing improvements in aerobic capacity, strength, endurance, body-mass index, balance, life satisfaction and quality of life.

As you now understand the wellness and preventative power of walking and fruit and vegetable consumption alone, you understand that these data represent significant decreases in susceptibility for developing cancer, heart disease, diabetes, depression, dementia, obesity, and every other chronic illness. You also understand what this behavior change means in terms of increased productivity, decreased absenteeism and presenteeism, and decreased healthcare costs. Most importantly, you understand what this means with respect to the health, vitality, and quality of life for the participants.

Summary:

Total Cups Of Water Consumed:	520,568
Average Cups Of Water/Person/Day:	6
Total Servings Of Fruits And Vegetables:	456,782
Average Daily Servings:	5.2

I don't think there is any better way for me to share my excitement and optimism than sharing some of the experiences of participants. Here are just a few examples. This is what makes all the hard work, all the travel, facing all the obstacles, and all the time worthwhile. This is the joy in what we do.

From a participant with Dr. Davy Rigsby
Rigsby Family Wellness Center - Jacksonville Texas:

"Thank you for your unconditional support!! Your enthusiasm and spirit are wonderfully infectious. Yesterday there was a blood drive at our church. The preacher announced that everyone who donated blood would get a free pint of ice cream!! Good grief! I was so happy to recognize what a poor life choice that makes. I was sad to think of this unhealthy offer! Have a great day and keep up the good work! You are making Jacksonville healthier everyday! That makes me smile!"

Donna

From a participant with Drs Marc and Colleen VanHoogstraat
Lifetime Wellness Family Chiropractic - Oxford, Michigan

"Today, August 1st, 2010, is one of the days in my life that should and believe me will be celebrated big time...I ran a complete mile this morning for the first time in my life...at 13.58 minutes the GREATEST time in the world, for me that is. Now all I have to do is beat my time and then go for two. I did this at the young age of 62 in just two weeks training/running and never running before in my whole life. Just think...if it wasn't for you guys, I would have given up with the first onset of shin splints ... I just love you both so much. Words you taught me that I now live by ... 'It is never too late to be what you might have been.' ... **I am now a real runner** ... Thank you, thank you, thank you so very much. Love you both."

Pamillia

Another participant with Drs Marc and Colleen VanHoogstraat
Lifetime Wellness Family Chiropractic Oxford - Michigan

This participant was in the very first graduating class of the Innate Lifestyle™ Program!

"Health has taken on a whole new meaning since going through the Innate Lifestyle Program. Through the Innate Lifestyle Program, I have learned to eat much better, move more and think about what's going on inside my head. Since last August when

I began this program with my husband, I have had a complete paradigm shift in how food, exercising and my thoughts directly relate to my overall health, energy and vitality.

I have learned so much. I have learned the effects of food on my body, both positive and negative. Prior to the Innate Lifestyle Program I had a lot of misinformation about food. I thought I was doing a lot of good things for myself and my family, and I was, but not what I am today after being educated about what our cells need to express health. It's very freeing to choose to eat fruits, vegetables, proteins, water and supplements when we know that's really all the food that our cells require to reflect health. The most amazing part of changing our paradigm about food is that our 3-year-old daughter has learned right along with us. What a blessing it is for her to begin at such a young age.

I have learned to gradually change my activity habits. I have learned to create at least two times in my day to stretch and get movement into my spine. I will be honest and say that at the beginning of the program I wasn't a very "athletic" person by doing things like running or using weights, but little by little I have learned how to work out and enjoy what I feel like afterwards. I have learned how exercise not only helps my body look physically better, but I have an increase in energy, I have a much better night's sleep and have a combatant towards stress each day. The program helped me keep track of my daily movement and guided me more on my individual progress.

Finally, the THINK WELL part of the Innate Lifestyle program was the most surprising to me. Surprising in that I had never realized how much my thought processes really affected my overall health. I have learned to begin each day with quiet time to keep myself centered and filled up with positives about myself. I have learned how my positive and negative self-talk effects my behaviors on a daily basis. I have learned strategies to focus on the sources of my emotions and behaviors. My belief systems and self-talk have changed greatly towards the better. My favorite part of THINK WELL is learning to love myself more and by doing this I can love my husband, daughter, family and friends better. It's stopping to reflect on the positives in my life and choosing to make the best of each moment. I am a different person today because of participating in the Innate Lifestyle Program.

The first time you mentioned the Innate Lifestyle Program to my husband and I, I was skeptical of spending the money and had doubts about starting a year long program. However, I realized that this was a great opportunity and a great way to change my family tree. I wanted a fresh start.

I wanted to be healthier. I wanted to move better. I wanted to think better. I wanted to make better choices for my family. I felt like I would regret not doing the Innate Lifestyle Program. My husband and I both wanted to make a change in our family. Having my husband doing the program alongside me was vitally important. We have grown so much together over the past year, supported each other when business got the better of us, and encouraged each other when we needed it. As a family, we've come away with a greater purpose for being the family God intended us to be, a love for eating healthy food, a desire to include movement into our everyday life, positive thinking and gratefulness for our many blessings. Thank you for being amazing coaches and mentors! Thank you for sharing all your gifts throughout this program."

From a participant with Dr. Michael Heinzlmeir
Pure Chiropractic - Red Deer, Alberta

"I started the Innate Lifestyle Program with the hope of becoming a happier and healthier person. With your support and encouragement as my lifestyle doctor and the gradual changes the program has asked me to make over the last few months I have seen tremendous changes in how I feel both physically and mentally. I have more energy than I have had for a long time and I am stronger and able to do things easier. I have opened myself up to actively participate in my health goals. My attitude towards myself has changed for the better. I am much nicer to myself. I am able to see and accept the victories I accomplish. I am making better food choices and I am learning to nourish my body, not feed my emotions. I am pleased with my recent assessment as it gave me evidence that I am getting healthier by making small positive changes in my behavior. I am grateful that I have had the opportunity to participate in the Innate Lifestyle Program and feel as I continue implementing healthier choices I am empowered to attain my goals."

M.M., female, age 51

From Dr. John Harper Harper
Chiropractic Wellness Center - Oceanside California

"Hello Dr. Chestnut, I want to thank you for the Innate Lifestyle Program, not just for my patients, but for myself. While I am in it for the long haul, in just two short months of adding the healthy behaviors of this program, I have experienced some wonderful changes.

The most obvious to me and others is my new calm demeanor. I now am able to handle life's ups and downs without frustration, anger or comfort foods. Situations that once would have "set me off" are now just part of the ebb and flow of the day. This has allowed me to be closer and more relaxed with those around me.

Another great change is my weight and associated symptoms. I have dropped 21 pounds from the combination of eating better and doing some moderate exercise. My previous diet was causing so much inflammation, that I had rather severe pitting edema in my legs. Today I have zero swelling and can readily see the veins in my feet again. I can only imagine the stress this was putting on my heart and vascular system.

I also have gained energy and the desire to do healthy behaviors. Eating fruit and vegetables used to be far down the list of desirable foods. Now my body craves these foods naturally like never before. Exercise used to be an event that I just detested. Now I look forward to my walks and the simple exercises recommended in the program.

The one improvement that I value the most, is that I just like myself better. I see these changes in my life as a way to gain some control over what seemed uncontrollable. Living a genetically congruent lifestyle is the greatest gift anyone can give to themselves and to their loved ones."

With deep gratitude, John

For your information here is the contact information for the licensed Eat Well Move Well Think Well Innate Lifestyle™ Program Centers:

Innate Lifestyle™ Program - Licensed Centers

Australia

1. Dr. Warren Genders, Belridge Chiropractic. 6/265 Eddystone Avenue, Beldon, Perth, WA 6027. (08) 9401 0777.
2. Healing Wave Chiropractic. 32 Queen Street, Warners Bay, NSW 2282. (61) 2 4948 4022.
3. Dr. Greg Kendall, 149 West Burleigh Road, Burleigh Heads, QLD 4220. 1330 39 69 89.
4. Dr. Andrew Mutzig, Shadowplay Pty. Ltd. 1 Flynn Street, Unit 10, Wembley, WA 6014. (61) 8 9388 0823.
5. Dr. Greg Parker, Northlakes Wellness Practice. 138 Wallarah Road, Gorokan NSW 2263. (02) 4392 1825.
6. Jeff Pow, Catalyst Wellness. PO Box 46, Leederville, WA 6007. (61) 4 1222 9564.
7. Dr. Wesley Upfold, Stirling Chiropractic Clinic. 569 Karrinyup Road, Stirling, WA 6021. (08) 9446 8322.

Canada

1. Dr. Richard Baxter and Dr. Adrian Raphael, Discover Chiropractic Family Wellness Centre. 16-1594 Fairfield Road, Victoria, BC V8S 1G1. 250-386-9355.
2. Dr. Shanna Frederick and Dr. Jenna Friesen, Frederick Family Chiropractic. Box 759, Watson, SK S0K 4V0. 306-287-4327.
3. Dr. Michael Heinzlmeir, Pure Lifestyle. 207-4807 50th Avenue, Red Deer, AB T4N 4A5. 403-348-8222.

4. Dr. Mark Hunter, Hunter Chiropractic Wellness Centre. 4380 Innes Road, Unit B, Ottawa, ON K4A 3W3. 613-841-9355.

5. Dr. Jeff Hindbo, LivWell Lifestyle Solutions. 4320 50th Avenue, Red Deer, AB T4N 3Z6. 403-373-5433.

6. Dr. Scott Macaulay, Macaulay Chiropractic Office and Wellness Lifestyle Center. 285 Bayfield Road, Goderich, ON N7A 3G8. 519-524-4104.

7. Dr. Raymond Roy, 3019 Pandosy Street, Kelowna, BC V1Y 1W3. 604-861-1332.

8. Dr. Jason Whittaker, Congruency Inc. 38 Proulx Place, Winnipeg, MB R4X 0C5. 204-282-7512.

United Kingdom

1. Dr. Stuart Lawrence, Body Active Services. 112 Rushbottom Lane, Benfleet, Essex, SS5 4RG. 0044 1268 752 123.

United States

1. Dr. Vlad Brajak, Advantage Family Chiropractic. 8023 W. Grand River Avenue, Suite 600, Brighton, MI 48114. 810-494-9300.

2. Dr. Tony Breitbach, Wellness Revolution. 1117 Emerson Street, Evanston, IL 60201. 847-869-1773.

3. Dr. David Butler, Century Chiropractic Center, 2308 S. Broadway, Suite 5, Alexandria, MN 56308. 320-762-0667.

4. Dr. Craig DeFries, WellAdjusted. 1810 30th Street, Suite E, Boulder, CO 80301. 303-447-3900.

5. Dr. Jamey Dyson, Advanced Chiropractic. 1295 Wallace Road NW, Salem, OR 97304. 503-361-3949.

6. Dr. Gary Harcourt, Innate-Wellness, LLC. 2670 Baker Street, York, PA 17408. 717-817-1656.

7. Dr. John Harper, Harper Chiropractic Wellness Center. 1816 Oceanside Blvd, Suite B, Oceanside, CA 92054. 760-722-3202.

8. Dr. Thomas Iacobelli, Align Wellness Center. 81 Railroad Place, Saratoga Springs, NY 12866. 518-682-2655.

9. Dr. Michael Johnson, Johnson Chiropractic. 2990 East Main Street, Richmond, IN 47374. 765-962-9900.

10. Dr. Arron R. Kalis, Innate Wellness Center, LLC. 220 South Main Street, Blue Earth, MN 56013. 507-526-2211.

11. Dr. Scott Lampshire and Florance O'Neal, M.S., L.C.P.C. Wellness Partners LLC. 725 6th Avenue East, Kalispell, MT 59901. 406-257-7572.

12. Dr. Keith Lavender, Foresight Chiropractic, PLC. 2915 E. Baseline Road, Suite 126. Gilbert, AZ 85234. 480-325-6977.

13. Dr. Jordan Leasure and Dr. Jade Leasure, North Shore Pro-Active Health. 112 W. Lake Street, Libertyville, IL 60048. 847-362-4476.

14. Dr. Joe Kelley and Yohko Kelley. LiveWell USA LLC. 12305 120th Avenue NE, Suite A, Kirkland, WA 98034. 425-820-2777.

15. Dr. Darrel Loder, Smoky Valley Chiropractic. 121 W. Lincoln, Lindsborg, KS 67456. 785-227-4455.

16. Dr. Staci Noyes. 2808 E 20th Street, Farmington, NM 87402. 505-327-9196.

17. Dr. Jason Omer, Omer Chiropractic Clinic, 501 SE Second Street, Washington, IN 47501. 812-254-0476.

18. Dr. Loyal Peterson, Peterson Family Chiropractic Wellness Center, 344 McDonald Street, Oconto, WI 54153. 920-834-2888.

19. Dr. Jonathan Rigsby, Rigsby Family Wellness Center, 307 W. Rusk Street, Jacksonville, TX 75766. 903-586-4460.

20. Dr. Sharla Robertson, Clearview Chiropractic Life Center. 5417 Acton Highway, Suite 101, Granbury, TX 76049. 817-326-1174.

21. Dr. Nick Sechrist, Merry Anne Sechrist, Barbara Mahoney, Center for Optimal Well-Being, LLC. 2505 Foresight Circle, Grand Junction, CO 81505. 970-270-6485.

22. Drs. Marc and Colleen VanHoogstraat, Lifetime Wellness Family Chiropractic. 51 S. Washington, Suite D, Oxford, MI 48371. 248-770-5616.

23. Drs. Amanda and Dennis Warren, Generations Chiropractic Wellness Center. 1422 North College Avenue, Fayetteville, AR 72703. 479-442-2755.

24. Dr. Cory Webb, Health First Wellness Center. 530 Madison Street, St. Charles, MO 63301. 636-946-3600.

25. Dr. Nicholas Wells, The Wellness Pointe Family Chiropractic. 16909 Burke Street, Suite 124, Omaha, NE 68118. 402-933-4463.

26. Dr. Jeffrey West, Be Truly Well Chiropractic & Day Spa. 19a Haines Street, Newark, DE 19711. 302-525-4343.

Chapter 13
Concluding Thoughts and Healthy Lifestyle Action Steps

"I have walked that long road to freedom. I have tried not to falter; I have made missteps along the way. But I have discovered the secret that after climbing a great hill, one only finds that there are many more hills to climb. I have taken a moment here to rest, to steal a view of the glorious vista that surrounds me, to look back on the distance I have come. But I can only rest for a moment, for with freedom come responsibilities, and I dare not linger, for my long walk is not ended."

Nelson Mandela

We have now answered the two most important questions facing our species. We have discovered that the reason humans are so sick with chronic illness, the reason humans are now the sickest species on the planet, is because we are making lifestyle choices, and creating and living in physical and social environments, that are genetically incongruent, that are chronically stressful. This chronic exposure to stressors causes the chronic genetic expression of alarm, stress, and adaptive physiology that is unsustainable and leads to fatigue, chronic illness, and early death. We are not sick due to pathological genes or pathological cell function, we are sick because we are living pathological lifestyles and living in pathological environments.

The research is unequivocal, chronic illness rates have increased exponentially over a few decades. This rapid increase in per capita chronic illness rates cannot be attributed to gene change as the human genome has remained virtually constant during this period. The rapid increase in per capita chronic illness rates cannot be attributed to aging because the rate of population aging is exponentially less than the rate of increase in chronic illness rates and, further, the most rapid rises in chronic illness rates are occurring among our children and middle aged populations. The rapid increase in per capita chronic illness rates cannot be attributed to increased diagnostic ability because the diagnostic tests for chronic illnesses like obesity and diabetes were available before the rapid per capita rises in these illnesses. Further, research shows that as non-industrial citizens adopt our lifestyle patterns they also rapidly develop the same chronic illnesses. We are not sick because of bad genes, bad cells, or bad luck; we are sick because of bad lifestyle choices.

This knowledge has allowed us to accurately answer the other most important question facing our species. We have learned that, as chronic illness is a lifestyle caused problem, the only viable solution to the chronic illness pandemic is changing lifestyle habits toward what is genetically congruent for our species.

In order to get and stay well, humans, like every other species, must eat, move, think, and interact in ways that our genome requires to express health and vitality.

Inside our genes is an innately intelligent and extraordinarily reliable recipe or blueprint for health and vitality. If we supply the right ingredients for this recipe or the right raw materials for this blueprint, the natural, inevitable result is the expression of health. Virtually every human being has the genetic potential for a long, happy life, whether we reach this potential is a product of our lifestyle choices. Even the vast minority of humans that do have genetically caused health issues have significantly greater health, and significantly greater quality of life, if they choose healthy versus unhealthy lifestyle choices.

Have humans become the sickest species on earth because of bad genes, bad cells, bad luck, or bad lifestyle choices?

No drug or surgery will ever be the solution for illness caused by deficient and/or toxic nutrition, deficient exercise or toxic postures, deficient and/or toxic thoughts and social interactions, or environmental toxins.

Both basic physiological, biochemical, and genetic science, as well as historical data, indicate that using drugs and surgery to change physiology and biochemistry has not been, and will never be, successful at restoring health or ever be a viable solution for wellness and prevention.

The only possible way to solve the chronic illness pandemic and the unsustainable economic and social burdens it is causing is to decrease the number of people developing chronic illness and to increase the number of people healing from chronic illness. In other words the only possible solution is fewer sick people or more healthy people. The only viable option for wellness and prevention is lifestyle change. Lifestyle intervention is the most evidence-based, most effective, and most cost-effective intervention.

This book has really been about answering WHY lifestyle is so important. I know that unless you know WHY changing your lifestyle is important you very likely will not make the effort to do so. If the reason for change or the reason for any particular choice does not matter to you then you just won't expend the effort and energy to do it. This is one of the great threats of the bad genes, bad cells, bad luck belief system. As I have mentioned repeatedly, if you don't believe lifestyle is the most significant factor determining why you are sick or whether you will get and stay well then lifestyle just won't matter to you.

I sincerely hope I have accomplished my goal of making lifestyle matter to you. My goal was to do just that. My goal was to make you understand and believe, beyond any reasonable doubt, that your lifestyle choices are the single most important factor determining your quality and quantity of life. I want you to understand that chronic illness is avoidable and that good health is attainable and that it is your responsibility to make the choices that determine your health destiny.

What is the single greatest determinant of human quality and quantity of life?

Now that you know WHY lifestyle choice is so important it is time to introduce information about WHAT lifestyle choices are required and HOW to empower yourself to make these choices. The book I am working on as you read this will contain great detail about what lifestyle choices are genetically congruent for the human species. The book will provide you with fascinating, in-depth and easily understood information regarding the eating, moving, thinking, and social interacting choices that you require to express your genetic potential for health and vitality. The book will also go into great detail about how to get yourself, and how to empower your loved ones, to make these choices – gradually, easily, comfortably, and sustainably.

Although I don't have the space for this detail in this book I do want to leave you with some information that you can immediately implement to improve your health and the health of your loved ones.

I want to begin by telling you that getting and staying well is not complicated and it is not difficult. You do not need to spend a lifetime sifting through the confusing misinformation about the necessity to find the right individual diet, exercise routine, or self help strategy for your unique genetic make-up, blood type, metabolic type, sex, age, race, hair color or hat size. The reason there are so many different "diets", exercise routines, and self help strategies is because nobody has asked or answered the right questions. Remember, your eating, moving, and thinking requirements are unique only to your species, not to you as an individual member of that species. Once you discover what the genetically required eating, moving, and thinking patterns are for the human species the confusion disappears.

I also want you to forget about all the times you have tried to change in the past without success. You did not fail, you got feedback. You did not get feedback that you are inherently weak or lazy or lacking willpower or incapable of change. You got feedback that the strategies you tried did not work. You tried to change your behaviors without changing your belief systems and that is just not sustainable.

What determines what behaviors we choose?

Behavior modification does not create sustainable change and it makes change unpleasant. Change is not hard, hard change is hard. Easy change is easy.

I teach easy change because it is the only change that works. If you believe that exercise is awful or that french fries are wonderful you will always behave accordingly. Trying to force yourself to stop doing what you enjoy and forcing yourself to do the things you dislike is miserable, it is just deprivation and nobody can sustain that. Your behaviors are logical based on your belief systems. It is your belief systems that are illogical.

Don't allow yourself to ever associate becoming healthier with deprivation or struggle. The fact is that nothing is more depriving or more of a struggle than being sick. Don't lie to yourself.

Getting healthy is not about struggling upstream against the current. Getting well is about floating downstream on an air mattress toward a beautiful paradise called health and vitality.

Remember, hard change is hard, easy change is easy. Use easy change to make healthy habits. Healthy habits are as hard to break as unhealthy ones. Healthy belief systems dictate healthy behaviors as easily and as naturally as unhealthy belief systems dictate unhealthy behaviors.

I have discovered that before you can expect change you have to teach people how to change. You can't just tell people what to do, you have to teach them how to get themselves to do it. I've learned the hard way that behavior modification doesn't work. You have to modify belief systems. You have to teach people that if they say, "I hate broccoli", they're not going to eat broccoli. If they say, "I hate exercise," it doesn't matter what you tell them, if they believe they hate exercise, they in fact hate exercise and they will take the logical steps to avoid it.

What is more depriving, being sick or avoiding the behavior patterns that make you sick?

One of the most important breakthroughs that I've had is that I have learned how to equip people with some information about how to assess, and then actively and successfully engage in changing, their belief systems. It is really about brain based learning. It is about moving away from punishment and reward (behavior modification) and moving toward matching belief systems to desired behaviors (belief system modification). It's not the old adage of "you can lead a horse to water but you can't make it drink" or "with the right system of reward and punishment we can make the horse drink". It is about learning how to make the horse realize or believe it is thirsty and thus create the natural thirst for water. It is indisputable that what people believe dictates their behavior. You can struggle for a short period of time to do what you don't like, or don't do what you do like, but in the end your behaviors always come back in line with your belief systems. Isn't this exactly what happens to you? You then blamed yourself. How tragic. You were not the problem, the advice you got was the problem.

It's not enough just to teach people what they should eat, and how they should move, and how they should think. It's that we have to teach them how to change their programming. We have to be able to teach them that it's not enough to wish for something consciously, they have to be able to dip into their belief systems, their subconscious belief systems, and reprogram those.

Everyone consciously "wants" to eat, move, and think better, they just don't realize that their subconscious beliefs are insurmountable obstacles undermining this wish.

When people learn how to choose healthy belief systems the potential is unlimited. Undeniably, your behaviors are the direct result of your beliefs and your subconscious programming. So, what you choose to eat is based on your subconscious programming, your belief systems. Whether you choose to exercise or choose not to exercise is based on how you feel about exercise, whether you associate something positive with exercise and something negative to not exercising, or whether you associate something positive with not exercising and something negative with exercising. This is true of all your behavior choices.

Are humans genetically programmed for a long, happy life or for a short, miserable existence? What is our true potential?

I will go into this in great detail in the next book, and this is an integral part of the Innate Lifestyle™ Program. For now I just want you to be aware that the reason you have not been successful at health or healthy behavior change in the past was not due to any inherent weaknesses you have. It was based on the inherent weaknesses of the strategies you were taught and your lack of the required, but very attainable, knowledge and skills you needed. You can't break the universal laws of belief system and behavior change and expect a good result.

You need to understand and accept the fact that you were born with all the innate ability you require to live a long, healthy, and happy life.

Regardless of where you are now, you have the ability to make some easy, comfortable changes that will produce a longer, better life for you.

You do not lack ability, you lack the proper information, coaching, practice, and support required to develop the proper skill set. Never question your ability and never tell yourself you are not capable. Always tell yourself the truth, that you are capable but that you just are not trained yet.

Start with this accurate belief system about yourself. You were born genetically beautiful and intelligent and capable and worthy of love and a joyful life. I mean real beauty, the kind that transcends superficial physical features. Have you ever met a happy, successful, loving and kind person that you found unattractive? Of course not, such a person does not exist. You may be unhealthy right now and the truth is that you may have changed your appearance for the worse with unhealthy lifestyle choices. You may have covered up your inner beauty but it is there; it never leaves you.

Don't think of change as becoming somebody else; think of change as returning to your wonderful, natural, gorgeous, capable self.

Can an unhealthy lifestyle choice cancel out the benefit of a healthy lifestyle choice? Is health an all or none concept?

Here is a list of things you can start doing right away. If any of these things makes you uncomfortable what should you do? Don't do them (yet) or simply modify them to make them comfortable.

1. **Add Positives First**: The first thing is that you must never begin any health program by taking away things that you like. This is just stressful and unpleasant. Always begin your journey toward better health, toward a better, longer life, by adding something healthy to your lifestyle. Find something that is healthy and that you either enjoy or don't mind doing and start there. You all have these things. The reason you are not doing them is because you have told yourself that there is no point doing the easy things if you are not going to do the hard things. You have the completely false belief system that if it is easy it is not beneficial or that the "bad" things you do would just cancel out any benefit. "No point going for a walk, I'm not giving up pizza or chocolate"."No point eating those extra helpings of vegetables, I just can't get myself to exercise." Health is not an all or none concept, every choice counts.

2. **Eat Fresh Fiber First**: One of the healthiest things you will ever do is eat more raw fruits and vegetables. Don't panic, I didn't say you had to eat a bowl full of brussel sprouts or broccoli everyday in order to get healthier. All you need

to do to increase your health from where it is right now is increase the amount of raw fruits and vegetables you are consuming. I call this my 'fresh fiber first' implementation step. Pick your favorite fruit or vegetable, I don't care what it is, and consume it more often. Make the effort to consume some form of raw fruit or vegetable with every meal or snack. If you only like grapes then make it grapes. It doesn't matter. What I can tell you is that if the only thing you changed in your lifestyle over the next year was to add a raw fruit or vegetable to every snack you would be significantly healthier in a year from now. Don't even think about anything else. Just find a fruit or vegetable that is EASY and COMFORTABLE to eat and eat it. I don't care if the meal or snack you consume it with is donuts or beer and pretzels or nachos. If you add the raw fruit or vegetable you get benefit.

If the only lifestyle change you made for the next year was to add raw fruits and vegetables to every meal and snack would you be healthier in a year from now?

3. **Take the Wellness and Prevention Paradigm Essential Supplements**: There are 4 supplements that the research unequivocally indicates are required for virtually every human living in industrial society. These are:

    Fish Oil: A natural EPA:DHA ratio, natural triglyceride form, full fatty acid complement fish oil for essential fatty acids (EPA and DHA).

    Vitamin D.

    Probiotic: A non-dairy, wheat free, soy free, multi-strain, probiotic that contains strains that are part of the normal human flora.

    Certified Organic Whole Food Micronutrient Formula: A certified organic, synthetic vitamin-free, whole food complex for vitamins and other essential micronutrients (phytochemicals, minerals, antioxidants).

    The best supplement is no supplement. However, there is virtually no way that you are going to be able to get sufficient intake of essential fatty acids or Vitamin D. You absolutely need to supplement with these. If you make your own fermented foods at home and consume them daily then you probably will not need a probiotic supplement. Similarly, if you consume a WIDE VARIETY of LOCAL, VINE-RIPENED, ORGANIC fruits and vegetables or if you make and consume your own vegetable juice with these organic vegetables on a daily basis you will probably not require the certified organic whole food supplement. For more information on why these supplements are required please go to www.innatechoice.com. There are newsletters, information videos, and a FAQ section that are free for you to access.

What is the best time of day to incorporate healthy physical activity into your daily routine?

4. **Incorporate Activity into your Work, Family and Social Life**: Start having events that involve activity with you and your family. If you're going to meet for coffee, meet a few minute walk from the coffee shop and walk together. There are so many things that we do which could easily involve activity. It is always more fun to go for a walk or do activity with somebody else. Go for family walks after dinner or in the morning. Play an active game with your kids. Play hide and seek, play tag, wrestle on the bed. Join an activity group or form one. Group dynamics are great, if you don't show up, they say, "hey, where were you yesterday?" Find something you ENJOY that involves physical movement and SCHEDULE time for it.

My advice is to schedule activity for first thing in the morning, it is the only time of day you have autonomy. There are too many uncontrolled variables after the day begins, do it first thing in the morning.

If you dread walking then would you be willing to just go outside for a few minutes and breath some fresh air to start your day? Now, I'm going to ask that you wear work-out clothes when you go outside. I'm not telling you to work out, I'm just asking if you would be willing to go outside, and when you're outside in your work-out clothes, if you would be willing to take some nice deep breaths. Are you comfortable with that? Would you also be willing to get your exercise clothes together and set them out before you go to bed the night before? Setting the clothes out programs your subconscious mind, and then you don't wake up and say, "I've got to get up;" you wake up and say, "I've got to go outside and breath in some fresh air." That's all I'm suggesting you do if that is all you are comfortable with. Eventually, you'll get so bored, what will you do? You'll walk. But I don't care if it takes you six months. It's not important. If you feel like it go for a walk, if you don't then just do your breathing and stretch if you feel like it. Make it easy, comfortable and gradual. Just developing the habit of getting up and getting exercise clothes on and going outside or to your exercise spot is HUGE. It is creating healthy habits.

5. **Always Shop Full**: No matter what, if you go to the supermarket and you're not full, eat before you shop for groceries. You are always better off to eat something, even if it's not great, to fill yourself up before you shop, because if you don't you'll wind up putting garbage into that cart or basket. I want you to know the battle is not won or lost at home; the battle is always won or lost at the point of purchase.

   Here's what I know about you. When you're at home and it's about 8:00 at night, and it's bon-bon time, and you're sitting in front of the television, you say to yourself, "I think I need a little something." If you go to the cupboard and it's not there, what will you do? You won't get in the car and go shopping will you? What will you do? You will search for an hour - all your secret spots. You'll search high and low until you are too exhausted or frustrated to continue. By the end of that search, you'll stagger into bed and fall asleep, and you'll wake up in the morning and say to yourself, "Well, I guess I didn't really need it, I'm actually glad I didn't eat it." If it's not in the house, you won't consume it. Very few people will get out of the house to go get it. Don't bring it home. I hear this argument all the time, "Well, my kids are going to get it out anyway." I don't care. Don't bring it in. If you don't bring it in your house, you won't eat it. And at the end of the day, no matter how bad that craving was, in the morning you'll be just fine; in fact you will be better off.

In terms of healthy food choices, where is the battle lost and won?

6. **Make Your Choices Based on how you will Feel After the Choice**: It's very important to get into the habit of judging your meal or whatever choice you're going to make by how you'll feel after, not before or during. How many of you have ever regretted a salad? "Oh, why did I eat that lettuce?" It doesn't happen. But how many of you have regretted unhealthy choices? All of you. You end up with three minutes of pleasure while you're engaging in the unhealthy choice and then you get what? Twenty-three hours and 57 minutes of guilt. So you need to pause and assess how you are going to feel after you eat the junkfood. Bring the thoughts about how you will feel after the choice to your conscious mind so they can compete with the thoughts about how you will feel during the choice. This will help you start to change some of those things, it is actually a first step in changing your belief systems about those choices.

Do you feel the same after making an unhealthy lifestyle choice as you do just before or during engaging in that unhealthy choice? Which feeling lasts longer and has the greatest impact on your quality of life?

7. **Start and End Everyday with Gratitude**: Every morning when you get up, before you get out of bed, take a moment and think about what you have to be grateful for that day. We all have something to be grateful for, even if it is the fact that we are alive and able to think at all. I would suggest that every one of you reading this have food and shelter and so many other things to be grateful for. I am not interested in debating whether or not you have troubles in your life. We all do. I'm only interested in pointing out two important facts. One, you have something to be grateful for. Two, reflecting on this will improve your health and improve your life and improve the lives of everyone you interact with.

   When you go to bed at night stop and pause to think about what you have to be grateful for regarding your day or your life in general. Tell your family members that they are safe and important and loved and appreciated. Always begin and end your day with gratitude. It is so easy. You don't even have to get out of bed to do it; you can just lie there and be grateful. If you do that every day for thirty days, do you know what will happen automatically when you open your eyes every morning? The first thought in your mind will be what? Gratitude. I promise it will. What a way to start each day. It changes everything.

I wrote my kids notes about how smart and handsome or beautiful, and brave, and kind, and honest they are. I wasn't sure how this would go over. Guess what they did? They taped them to their headboards and I have been reading them every night since! I also sing them a song every night that includes words about having a happy sleep and how I have loved them more each day since they were born. They won't go to sleep without it now. I also regularly tell them how safe, loved and important they are. I tell them that they have champion's hearts and scientist's minds.

Please do this for your children. Feed them good foods, feed them healthy movement and play, and feed them love and confidence and self esteem. Do the same for your spouses and other loved ones in your life.

Take time each day to tell people that they are loved and important and appreciated and tell them exactly why they are loved and important. Make them feel safe about your relationship with them. Feeling safe comes from being able to trust. Be trustworthy and be kind and be forgiving; of yourself and of others.

What is the first thing you should do every morning and the last thing you should do every night?

Life is such a gift. In terms of the age of the universe, or even the age of the earth, or the amount of time there has been life on earth, our human lifespan is a blink. Of all the options in the universe, it is beyond comprehension that the atoms that make up your body and mind have come together to allow you to consciously experience and appreciate life. Every choice we make that unnecessarily reduces our quantity or quality of life, or the quantity and quality of life of others, is an affront.

Embrace this gift of life and extract every ounce of enjoyment out of it. That is the purpose of your existence; to extract, and help others extract, every possible ounce of joy.

The single greatest determinant of your ability to do this is your health. The single greatest determinant of your health is your lifestyle; how you eat, move, think, and interact. Your genes contain the recipe or the blueprint regarding what is required in terms of your lifestyle to express your potential for health and happiness and thus extract the most joy out of your existence on earth. Don't commit suicide with your lifestyle choices. Follow your genetic recipe and supply the right lifestyle ingredients; commit constant acts of self preservation and self empowerment and role model this way of life for others.

"Our deepest fear is not that we are inadequate. Our deepest fear is that we are powerful beyond measure. It is our light, not our darkness that most frightens us. We ask ourselves, 'Who am I to be brilliant, gorgeous, talented and fabulous?' Actually, who are you not to be? You are a child of the universe; your playing small doesn't serve the world. There's nothing enlightened about shrinking so other people won't feel insecure around you. We are born to make manifest the glory of all that's within us. It's not just in some of us, it's in everyone. And as we let our light shine, we unconsciously give other people permission to do the same. As we are liberated from our own fear, our presence automatically liberates others."

Why have humans become so sick with chronic illness? What do we need to do to get and stay well?

Marianne Williamson

Welcome to the Wellness & Prevention Paradigm. Life is healthier and more joyful here. You belong here and you are welcome.

Create an extraordinary life.

With love and appreciation,

James

Endnotes

[1] Eaton et al., in Stone Agers in the Fast Lane: Chronic Degenerative Diseases In Evolutionary Perspective. (1988), pp. 739-749.

[2] "Partnership to Fight Chronic Disease," Almanac of Chronic Disease, (2009)

[3] Collins JJ, Baase CM, Sharda CE, et al. "The assessment of chronic health conditions on work performance, absence, and total economic impact for employers," Journal of Occupational and Environmental Medicine. (2005) pp. 547-557.

[4] "Partnership to Fight Chronic Disease," Almanac of Chronic Disease, (2009)

[5] U.S. Summary Tape File 3 for 1990 census data, and Summary File 4 and Census 2000 special tabulations for Census 2000 data.

[6] "Partnership to Fight Chronic Disease," Almanac of Chronic Disease, (2009)

[7] Eaton SB, & Cordain L., Evolutionary health promotion. Prev Med 2002; 34:109-118.

[8] Wu, Shin-Yi and Anthony Green. Projection of Chronic Illness Prevalence and Cost Inflation. RAND Corporation. October 2000.

[9] Medicare Current Beneficiary Survey/Families USA Foundation

[10] Paulette C. Morgan, "CRS Report for Congress," Health Care Spending: Past trends and projections. (2004)

[11] Houlihan J, Kropp T, Wiles R, Gray S, Campbell C, et al. Body burden: the pollution in newborns. Washington, DC: Environmental Working Group; July 14, 2005.

[12] Mark A. Hyman, MD; Dean Ornish, MD; Michael Roizen, MD, "Lifestyle Medicine: Treating The Causes Of Disease," Alternative Therapies, Nov/ Dec 2010

[13] Sterling, Peter in Schulkin, Jay. (2004)Allostasis, Homeostasis, and the Costs of Physiological Adaptation. Cambridge University Press, Cambridge U.K.

[14] Katharine Greider, The Big Fix: How the Pharmaceutical Industry Rips Off American Consumers, Public Affairs, 2003..

[15] Thomas S. Kuhn, The Structure of Scientific Revolutions (1962) publ. University of Chicago Press, 1962

[16] George Bernard Shaw, Man and Superman (1903)

[17] Linder J, and Stafford RS. Antibiotic treatment of adults with sore throat by primary care physicians: a national survey, 1989-1999. JAMA. 2001 Sep 12; 286(10):1181-6.

[18] Vastag B. Pay attention: ritalin acts much like cocaine. JAMA . 2001 Aug 22-29;286(8):905-6

[19] Magno Zito J et.al. Trends in Prescribing Psychotropic Medications to Preschoolers. JAMA . 2000;283:1025-1030.

[20] Conquering Suffering, Enriching Humanity, The World Heath Report' – World Health Organization, Geneva 1997

[21] Ibid.

[22] Roberts, C.K. & Barnard, J.B. Effects of exercise and diet on chronic disease. 2005 J. Appl Physiol 98 3-30.

[23] Ibid.

[24] Eaton et al. Stone agers in the fast lane: Chronic degenerative diseases in evolutionary perspective. 1988; Am. J. Med. 84, 739-749

[25] Ibid.

[26] Lichtenstein P, Holm NV, Verkasalo PK, Iliadou A,Kaprio J, Koskenvuo M, Pukkala E, Skytthe A, and Hemminki K. Environmental and heritable factors in the causation of cancer—analyses of cohorts of twins from Sweden, Denmark,and Finland. N Engl J Med 343: 78–85, 2000

[27] Hu FB, Manson JE, Stampfer MJ, Colditz G, Liu S, Solomon CG, and Willett WC. Diet, lifestyle, and the risk of type 2 diabetes mellitus in women. N Engl J Med 345: 790–797,2001.

[28] Stampfer MJ, Hu FB, Manson JE, Rimm EB, and Willett WC. Primary prevention of coronary heart disease in women through diet and lifestyle. N Engl J Med 343: 16–22, 2000.

[29] Eaton SB, Strassman BI, Nesse RM, Neel JV, Ewald PW, Williams GC, Weder AB, Eaton SB 3rd, Lindeberg S, Konner MJ, Mysterud I, Cordain L. Evolutionary health promotion. Prev Med 2002; 34:109-118.

[30] Eaton, Cordain & Lindeberg. Evolutionary Health Promotion: A Consideration of Common Counterarguments. Preventive Medicine 2002 (34) 119-123

[31] Partnership to Fight Chronic Disease," Almanac of Chronic Disease, (2009)

[32] Rippe J. Lifestyle Medicine and Health Care Reform. Am J Lifestyle Med. Nov/Dec 2009

[33] Watters, Ethan. DNA is not Destiny: The New Science of Epigenetics Rewrites the Rules of Disease, Heredity, and Identity. Discover Nov 2006

[34] Ibid.

[35] Ibid.

[36] Ibid.

[37] Ibid.

[38] Sorensen, et al. Genetic and Environmental Influence on Premature Death in Adult Adoptees. New England Journal of Medicine 318(1988): 727-32

[39] Lichtenstein et al. Environmental and Heritable Factors in the Causation of Cancer – Analyses of Cohorts of Twins from Sweden, Denmark, and Finland. New England Journal of Medicine 343, no. 2 (2000): 78-85

[40] Cao L, et.al. Environmental and Genetic Activation of a Brain-Adipocyte BDNF/Leptin Axis Causes Cancer Remission and Inhibition. Cell. 2010 Jul 9;142(1):52-64.

[41] Lipton, Bruce. The Biology of Belief Elite Books Santa Rosa CA, U.S.A. 2005

[42] Willet, W.C. (2002) Balancing Lifestyle and Genomics Research for Disease Prevention. Science 296: 695-698

[43] Selye, H. The Stress of Life. 1978. McGraw Hill.

[44] Epel, E.S. et al. Dec. 7, 2004 Accelerated telomere shortening in response to life stress. PNAS 101(49); 17312-17315

[45] Dhabhar, F. S. and McEwen, B. S. Moderate stress enhances, and chronic stress suppresses, cell-mediated immunity in vivo. Abstracts, Soc. Neurosci. 22, #536.3-p 1350. 96.

[46] Guyton, Arthur C. Textbook of Medical Physiology, 8th edition. 1991. W.B. Saunders. Philadelphia, PA, USA

[47] Markowe, H. L. J., M. G. Marmot, M. J. Shipley, C. J. Bulpitt, T. W. Meade, Y. Stirling, M. V. Vickers, and A. Semmence. Fibrinogen: a possible link between social class and coronary heart disease. Brit.Med.Jnl 291: 1312-1314,1985.

[48] Quirarte, G. L., B. Roozendaal, and J. L. McGaugh. Glucocorticoid enhancement of memory storage involves noradrenergic activation in the basolateral amygdala. Proc.Natl.acad.Sci.USA 94: 14048-14053, 1997

[49] McEwen, Bruce. Central effects of stress hormones in health and disease: understanding the protective and damaging effects of stress and stress mediators. Eur J Pharmacol. 2008 April 7; 583(2-3): 174–185.

[50] Michael Meaney Ph.D. Stress and Disease: Who Gets Sick: Who Stays Well Cortext Educational Seminars 2001

[51] McEwen, B. S. Stress and hippocampal plasticity. Annu.Rev.Neurosci. 22: 105-122, 1999. AND McEwen, B. S. Possible mechanisms for atrophy of the human hippocampus. Molecular Psychiatry 2: 255-262, 1997.

[52] Seeman, T. E., B. S. McEwen, B. H. Singer, M. S. Albert, and J. W. Rowe. Increase in Urinary Cortisol Excretion and Memory Declines: MacArthur Studies of Successful Aging. J.Clin.Endocrinol.Metab. 82: 2458-2465, 1997.

[53] Rockwood K. Physical activity and risk of cognitive impairment and dementia in elderly persons. Arch Neurol 58: 498–504, 2001.

[54] Marshall, D.A. et al. Optimal healing environments for chronic cardiovascular disease. J Altern Complement Med. 2004; 10 Suppl 1:S147-55

[55] Gilbert, M. Weaving Medicine Back Together: Mind-Body Medicine in the Twenty-First Century 2003 J. of Alt and Compl Med 9 (4).

[56] Van Cauter, E., K. S. Polonsky, and A. J. Scheen. Roles of circadian rhythmicity and sleep in human glucose regulation. Endocr.Rev. 18: 716-738, 1997.

[57] Esch, T. et al. The role of stress in neurodegenerative diseases and mental disorders. Neuro Endocrinol Lett. 2002 June; 23(3):199-208

[58] Brindley, D. N. and Y. Rolland. Possible connections between stress, diabetes, obesity, hypertension and altered lipoprotein metabolism that may result in atherosclerosis. Clin.Science 77: 453-461, 1989.

[59] Ibid.

[60] Shrivastava et al. Chronic cholesterol depletion using statins impairs the function and dynamics of human serotonin receptors. Biochemistry 2010 49 (26): 5426-5435

[61] Executive Summary of the Third Report of the National Cholesterol Education Program (NCEP) Expert Panel on Detection, Evaluation, and Treatment of High Blood Cholesterol in Adults (Adult Treatment Panel III). JAMA, 2001:285 (19): 2486-2497

[62] Abramson, John. (2004) Overdosed America: The Broken Promise of American Medicine. Harper Collins Inc. New York, New York, U.S.A.

[63] Ibid.

[64] Kjaergaard, et al. (2009) Low occurrence of ishemic heart disease among Inuit around 1963 suggested from ECG among 1851 East Greenland Inuit. Atherosclerosis, 203 (2); 599-603

[65] Cordain, L. Cereal Grains: Humanity's Double Edged Sword in Simopoulous, AP (ed): Evolutionary Aspects of Nutrition and Health. Diet, Exercise, Genetics and Chronic Disease. World Rev Nutr Diet. Basel, Karger, 1999, vol 84, pp19-73

[66] Pollan, Michael. 2006. The Omnivore's Dilemma: A Natural History of Four Meals. The Penguin Press.

[67] New, S.A. "Dietary influences on bone mass and bone metabolism: further evidence of a positive link between fruit and vegetable consumption and bone health? Am J Clin Nutr 2000; 71:142-151

[68] Seaman D. Health care for our bones: a practical nutritional approach to preventing osteoporosis. J Manipulative Physiol Ther. 2004 Nov-Dec; 27 (9) :591-5. PubMed PMID:15614247.

[69] U.S. National Institutes of Health 2000. John Hopkins Bayview Medical Center

[70] Seeman, T. E., B. H. Singer, J. W. Rowe, R. I. Horwitz, and B. S. McEwen. Price of adaptation --allostatic load and its health consequences: MacArthur studies of successful aging. Arch Intern Med 157: 2259-2268, 1997.

[71] Degner et al. Severe adverse drug reactions of antidepressants: results of the German multicenter drug surveillance program AMSP. Pharmacopsychiatry March 2004 37; Suppl 1: S39-45

[72] Fournier et al. (2010) Antidepressant Drug Effects and Depression Severity. JAMA 303 (1): 47-53

[73] Wu, Shin-Yi and Green, Anthony. Projection of Chronic Illness Prevalence and Cost Inflation. RAND Corporation, Oct. 2000.

[74] U.S. National Institutes of Health, 2000 John Hopkins Bayview Medical Center

[75] Almanac of Chronic Disease, 2009 Partnership to Fight Chronic Disease

[76] Eric A. Finkelstein, Justin G. Trogdon, Joel W. Cohen, and William Dietz. "Annual Medical Spending Attributable To Obesity: Payer- And Service-Specific Estimates."AND American Heart Association 2010

[77] American Diabetes Association 2010

[78] American Cancer Society 2010

[79] Siris, E.S. et al. Identification adn fracture outcomes of undiagnosed low bone mineral density in postmenopausal women. Results from the national oseoporosis risk assessment. J Am Med Assoc 2001;74:571-573

[80] CRS Report for Congress. Health Care Spending: Past trends and projections. (Updated April 8, 2004)

[81] Booth FW, Gordon SE, Carlson CJ, Hamilton MT. Waging war on modern chronic diseases: primary prevention through exercise biology. J Appl Physiol. 2000 Feb; 88 (2) :774-87. PubMed PMID:10658050.

[82] Rippe J. Lifestyle Medicine and Health Care Reform. Am J Lifestyle Med. Nov/Dec 2009

[83] Kilo & Larson. 2009. Exploring the harmful effects of health care. JAMA Vol 302: No 1.

[84] Ibid.

[85] Partnership to Fight Chronic Disease. 2009 Almanac of Chronic Disease.

[86] Hyman MA, Ornish D, Roizen M. Lifestyle medicine: treating the causes of disease. Alternative Therapies in Health and Medicine. 2009 Nov-Dec; 15 (6) :12-4. PubMed PMID:19943572.

[87] Ibid.

[88] Ibid.

[89] Ibid

[90] Ibid.

[91] Ibid.

[92] Ibid.

[93] Ibid.

[94] Ibid.

[95] The Power of Prevention: Chronic disease…the public health challenge of the 21st century. National Center for Chronic Disease Prevention and Health Promotion 2009.

[96] Ornish D, Magbanua MJ, Weidner G, Weinberg V, Kemp C, Green C, Mattie MD, Marlin R, Simko J, Shinohara K, Haqq CM, Carroll PR. Changes in prostate gene expression in men undergoing an intensive nutrition and lifestyle intervention. Proc Natl Acad Sci U S A. 2008 Jun 17; 105 (24) :8369-74. PubMed PMID:18559852; PubMed Central PMCID: PMC2430265.

[97] Ibid.

[98] Roberts, C.K. & Barnard, J.B. Effects of exercise and diet on chronic disease. 2005 J. Appl Physiol 98 3-30.

[99] Booth et al. Waging war on physical inactivity: using modern molecular ammunition against an ancient enemy J Appl Physiol 93: 3-30, 2002

[100] Hertog, MG. et al. Fruit and vegetable consumption and cancer mortality. Cancer Epidemiology, Biomarkers & Prevention. 1996 Vol. 5;9:673-677.

[101] Power of Prevention: Chronic disease…the public health challenge of the 21st century document. National Center for Chronic Disease Prevention and Health Promotion 2009

[102] The 2009 Almanac of Chronic Disease. Partnership to Fight Chronic Disease. 2009

[103] Ibid.

[104] Proof Positive: An Analysis of the Cost-Effectiveness of Worksite

Wellness, Summex Health Management, 2005

[105] Chestnut, J.L. 2003. The 14 Foundational Premises for the Scientific and Philosophical Validation of the Chiropractic Wellness Paradigm. The Wellness Practice – Global Self Health Corp. Victoria, BC., Canada.

[106] Ibid.

[107] Eric Jensen. Brain-Based Learning. The Brain Store 1995 San Diego, CA USA

[108] Jensen, E. 2000 Brain-Based Learning: The New Science of Teaching and Training. The Brain Store, San Diego, CA USA

[109] Seaman, D.R. Dysafferentation: a novel term to describe the neurophysiological effects of joint complex dysfunction. A look at likely mechanisms of symptom generation. J Manip Physiol Ther 1998;21 (4)

[110] Ibid.

[111] Videman, T. Experimental models of osteoarthritis: the role of immobilization. Clinical Biomechanics 1987 (2)

[112] Seaman, D.R. Dysafferentation: a novel term to describe the neurophysiological effects of joint complex dysfunction. A look at likely mechanisms of symptom generation. J Manip Physiol Ther 1998;21 (4)

[113] Ibid.

[114] Terret et al. Manipulation and pain tolerance. American Journal of Physical Medicine 1984 63 (5)

[115] Dr. Hayek, Ph.D 9th International Conference on Spinal Manipulation Oct 5, 2002 Reported in Advance 23 (2) Foundation for Chiropractic Education and Research

[116] Tuchin, Peter J. The effect of chiropractic spinal manipulative therapy on salivary cortisol levels. Journal of the Academy of Chiropractic Orthopedists 7 (2) July 1998

[117] Whitingham, W & Nilsson, N. Active range of motion in the cervical spine increases after spinal manipulation. J of Manip Physiol Ther 2001 24 (9)

[118] Haavik-Taylor, H. & Murphy, B. Cervical spine manipulation alters sensorimotor integration: A somatosensory evoked potential study. Clinical Neurophysiology 118 (2007) 391-402

[119] Wilk v. American Medical Association, (7th Cir. 1990)

[120] Ibid.

[121] Ibid.

[122] Manga, P. et al. A study to examine the effectiveness and cost-effectiveness of chiropractic management of low-back pain. 1993 Kenilworth Publishing, Ontario, Canada. Funded by the Ontario Ministry of Health.

[123] Ibid.

[124] Ibid.

[125] Norris JW, Beletsky V, Nadareishvili ZG. Sudden neck movement and cervical artery dissection. The Canadian Stroke Consortium. CMAJ 2000;163:38-40.

[126] Canadian Chiropractic Association. Reported testimony of Dr. J.W. Norris. In: Chiropractic Communications Working Group Information Bulletin; June 18, 2002. p. 2-40. Available at http://www.ccachiro.org.

[127] Chestnut, J.L. The Stroke Issue: Paucity of Valid Data, Plethora of Unsubstantiated Conjecture. J Manipulative Physiol Ther June 2004 27 (5) 368-372

[128] Ibid.

[129] Symons BP, Leonard T, Herzog W. Internal forces sustained by the vertebral artery during spinal manipulative therapy. J Manipulative Physiol Ther 2002;25:504-510.

Bibliography

- A Healthier Future For All Australians – Final Report of the National Health and Hospitals Reform Commission – June 2009 © Commonwealth of Australia, 2009
- CRS Report for Congress. Health Care Spending: Past trends and projections. (Updated April 8, 2004) Paulette C. Morgan.
- Executive Summary of the Third Report of the National Cholesterol Education Program (NCEP) Expert Panel on Detection, Evaluation, and Treatment of High Blood Cholesterol in Adults (Adult Treatment Panel III). JAMA, 2001:285 (19): 2486-2497.
- The 2009 Almanac of Chronic Disease. Partnership to Fight Chronic Disease.
- The Center for Disease Control 2008 National Ambulatory Medical Care Survey.
- The World Health Report 1997--conquering suffering, enriching humanity. World Health Forum. 1997; 18 (3-4) :248-60. PubMed PMID:9478137.
- Proceedings of the International Conference on the Return of Omega 3 Fatty Acids into the Food Supply I Land-Based Animal Food Products Bethesda, Maryland, USA September 18-19, 1997. World Rev Nutr Diet. 1998; 83:IX-XII, 1-240. PubMed PMID:9679023.
- The fifth report of the Joint National Committee on Detection, Evaluation, and Treatment of High Blood Pressure (JNC V). Arch Intern Med. 1993 Jan 25; 153 (2) :154-83. PubMed PMID:8422206.
- The Ninth International Conference on Spinal Manipulation Oct 5, 2002 Toronto - Reported in FCER Advance 23 (2)

- Abbott S, Trinkaus E, Burr DB. Dynamic bone remodeling in later Pleistocene fossil hominids. Am J Phys Anthropol. 1996 Apr; 99 (4) :585-601. PubMed PMID:8779340.
- Abramson, John. Overdosed America: The Broken Promise of American Medicine. Harper Collins Publishers Inc. New York, NY. 2004.
- Ader, R., 'Behavioural conditioning and the immune system' in Temoshok, L., Van Dyke, C., and Zegans, L. (eds), Emotions in Health and Illness, Gruner and Stratton, 1983.
- Akin F, Bastemir M, Alkis E. Effect of insulin sensitivity on SHBG levels in premenopausal versus postmenopausal obese women. Adv Ther. 2007 Nov-Dec; 24 (6) :1210-20. PubMed PMID:18165203.
- Alley DE, Crimmins E, Bandeen-Roche K, Guralnik J, Ferrucci L. Three-year change in inflammatory markers in elderly people and mortality: the Invecchiare in Chianti study. J Am Geriatr Soc. 2007 Nov; 55 (11) :1801-7. PubMed PMID:17727645; PubMed Central PMCID: PMC2646097.
- Alm JS, Swartz J, Lilja G, Scheynius A, Pershagen G. Atopy in children of families with an anthroposophic lifestyle. Lancet. 1999 May 1; 353 (9163) :1485-8. PubMed PMID:10232315.
- Allen, JM. The effects of chiropractic care on the immune system: A review of the literature. Chiropractic Journal of Australia 1993
- Althuis MD, Dozier JM, Anderson WF, Devesa SS, Brinton LA. Global trends in breast cancer incidence and mortality 1973-1997. Int J Epidemiol. 2005 Apr; 34 (2) :405-12. PubMed PMID:15737977.
- Archer SL, Liu K, Dyer AR, Ruth KJ, Jacobs DR Jr, Van Horn L, Hilner JE, Savage PJ. Relationship between changes in dietary sucrose and high density lipoprotein cholesterol: the CARDIA study Coronary Artery Risk Development in Young Adults. Ann Epidemiol. 1998 Oct; 8 (7) :433-8. PubMed PMID:9738689.
- Armaiz-Pena GN, Lutgendorf SK, Cole SW, Sood AK. Neuroendocrine modulation of cancer progression. Brain Behav Immun. 2009 Jan; 23 (1) :10-5. PubMed PMID:18638541; PubMed Central PMCID: PMC2630522.
- Atrens DM. The questionable wisdom of a low-fat diet and cholesterol reduction. Soc Sci Med. 1994 Aug; 39 (3) :433-47. PubMed PMID:7939861.

- Badyaev AV. Stress-induced variation in evolution: from behavioural plasticity to genetic assimilation. Proc Biol Sci. 2005 May 7; 272 (1566) :877-86. PubMed PMID:16024341; PubMed Central PMCID: PMC1564094.
- Bang HO, Dyerberg J. Lipid metabolism and ischemic heart disease in Greenland Eskimos. In: Draper HH, editor. Advances in nutrition research. New York: Plenum Publishing; 1980. p. 1-22.
- Banks WE, d'Errico F, Peterson AT, Kageyama M, Sima A, Sánchez-Goñi MF. Neanderthal extinction by competitive exclusion. PLoS One. 2008; 3 (12) :e3972. PubMed PMID:19107186; PubMed Central PMCID: PMC2600607.
- Baranzini SE, Mudge J, van Velkinburgh JC, Khankhanian P, Khrebtukova I, Miller NA, Zhang L, Farmer AD, Bell CJ, Kim RW, May GD, Woodward JE, Caillier SJ, McElroy JP, Gomez R, Pando MJ, Clendenen LE, Ganusova EE, Schilkey FD, Ramaraj T, Khan OA, Huntley JJ, Luo S, Kwok PY, Wu TD, Schroth GP, Oksenberg JR, Hauser SL, Kingsmore SF. Genome, epigenome and RNA sequences of monozygotic twins discordant for multiple sclerosis. Nature. 2010 Apr 29; 464 (7293) :1351-6. PubMed PMID:20428171; PubMed Central PMCID: PMC2862593.
- Barefield, Eric. Osteoporosis-Related Hip Fractures Cost $13 Billion to $18 Billion Yearly. USDA.gov Publications – Moving Towards Healthier Diets. Jan – April 1996.
- Barnard RJ, Jung T, Inkeles SB. Diet and exercise in the treatment of NIDDM The need for early emphasis. Diabetes Care. 1994 Dec; 17 (12) :1469-72. PubMed PMID:7882819.
- Barnard RJ, Aronson WJ. Preclinical models relevant to diet, exercise, and cancer risk. Recent Results Cancer Res. 2005; 166:47-61. PubMed PMID:15648182.
- Befus AD, Mathison R, Davison J. Integration of neuro-endocrine immune responses in defense of mucosal surfaces. Am J Trop Med Hyg. 1999 Apr; 60 (4 Suppl) :26-34. PubMed PMID:10344674.
- Begley S. The sins of the fathers, take 2. Newsweek. 2009 Jan 26; 153 (4) :18. PubMed PMID:19209517.
- Bellingrath S, Weigl T, Kudielka BM. Chronic work stress and exhaustion

is associated with higher allostastic load in female school teachers. Stress. 2009; 12 (1) :37-48. PubMed PMID:18951244.

- Benson, H. 1996. Timeless Healing: The Power and Biology of Belief. Fireside. New York, NY.
- Bengmark S. Immunonutrition: role of biosurfactants, fiber, and probiotic bacteria. Nutrition. 1998 Jul-Aug; 14 (7-8) :585-94. PubMed PMID:9684261.
- Benson, Herbert. The Relaxation Response. 1975 William and Morrow Inc. New York, NY.
- Berkman LF, Seeman T. The influence of social relationships on aging and the development of cardiovascular disease--a review. Postgrad Med J. 1986 Aug; 62 (730) :805-7. PubMed PMID:3774718; PubMed Central PMCID: PMC2418818.
- Best R, Lewis DA, Nasser N. The anti-ulcerogenic activity of the unripe plantain banana (Musa species). Br J Pharmacol. 1984 May; 82 (1) :107-16. PubMed PMID:6329384; PubMed Central PMCID: PMC1987262.
- Billman GE. Aerobic exercise conditioning: a nonpharmacological antiarrhythmic intervention. J Appl Physiol. 2002 Feb; 92 (2) :446-54. PubMed PMID:11796650.
- Blair SN, LaMonte MJ, Nichaman MZ. The evolution of physical activity recommendations: how much is enough?. Am J Clin Nutr. 2004 May; 79 (5) :913S-920S. PubMed PMID:15113739.
- Booth FW, Chakravarthy MV, Gordon SE, Spangenburg EE. Waging war on physical inactivity: using modern molecular ammunition against an ancient enemy. J Appl Physiol. 2002 Jul; 93 (1) :3-30. PubMed PMID:12070181.
- Booth FW, Chakravarthy MV, Spangenburg EE. Exercise and gene expression: physiological regulation of the human genome through physical activity. J Physiol. 2002 Sep 1; 543 (Pt 2) :399-411. PubMed PMID:12205177; PubMed Central PMCID: PMC2290514.
- Booth FW, Gordon SE, Carlson CJ, Hamilton MT. Waging war on modern chronic diseases: primary prevention through exercise biology. J Appl Physiol. 2000 Feb; 88 (2) :774-87. PubMed PMID:10658050.

- Borgman RF. Dietary factors in essential hypertension. Prog Food Nutr Sci. 1985; 9 (1-2) :109-47. PubMed PMID:3003794.
- Boyd-Woschinko G, Kushner H, Falkner B. Androgen excess is associated with insulin resistance and the development of diabetes in African American women. J Cardiometab Syndr. 2007 Fall; 2 (4) :254-9. PubMed PMID:18059208.
- Brach JS, Simonsick EM, Kritchevsky S, Yaffe K, Newman AB, Health, Aging and Body Composition Study Research Group. The association between physical function and lifestyle activity and exercise in the health, aging and body composition study. J Am Geriatr Soc. 2004 Apr; 52 (4) :502-9. PubMed PMID:15066063.
- Braun BL. Postural differences between asymptomatic men and women and craniofacial pain patients. Arch Phys Med Rehabil. 1991 Aug; 72 (9) :653-6. PubMed PMID:1859260.
- Braun BL, Amundson LR. Quantitative assessment of head and shoulder posture. Arch Phys Med Rehabil. 1989 Apr; 70 (4) :322-9. PubMed PMID:2930348.
- Bravi F, Edefonti V, Bosetti C, Talamini R, Montella M, Giacosa A, Franceschi S, Negri E, Ferraroni M, La Vecchia C, Decarli A. Nutrient dietary patterns and the risk of colorectal cancer: a case-control study from Italy. Cancer Causes Control. 2010 Nov; 21 (11) :1911-8. PubMed PMID:20680437.
- Brennan PC, Kokjohn K, Kaltinger CJ, Lohr GE, Glendening C, Hondras MA, McGregor M, Triano JJ. Enhanced phagocytic cell respiratory burst induced by spinal manipulation: potential role of substance P. J Manipulative Physiol Ther. 1991 Sep; 14 (7) :399-408. PubMed PMID:1719112.
- Brennan PC, Triano JJ, McGregor M, Kokjohn K, Hondras MA, Brennan DC. Enhanced neutrophil respiratory burst as a biological marker for manipulation forces: duration of the effect and association with substance P and tumor necrosis factor. J Manipulative Physiol Ther. 1992 Feb; 15 (2) :83-9. PubMed PMID:1373431.
- Bribiescas RG, Hickey MS. Population variation and differences in serum leptin independent of adiposity: a comparison of Ache Amerindian men of Paraguay and lean American male distance runners.

Nutr Metab (Lond). 2006 Aug 30; 3:34. PubMed PMID:16942616; PubMed Central PMCID: PMC1564401.

- Brown S, Martinez MJ, Parsons LM. The neural basis of human dance. Cereb Cortex. 2006 Aug; 16 (8) :1157-67. PubMed PMID:16221923.
- Brownell KD, Warner KE. The perils of ignoring history: Big Tobacco played dirty and millions died How similar is Big Food?. Milbank Q. 2009 Mar; 87 (1) :259-94. PubMed PMID:19298423.
- Bryson, B. 2003. A Short History of Nearly Everything. Transworld Publishers. London.
- Burstein E, Fearon ER. Colitis and cancer: a tale of inflammatory cells and their cytokines. J Clin Invest. 2008 Feb; 118 (2) :464-7. PubMed PMID:18219390; PubMed Central PMCID: PMC2213379.
- Cameron OG. Visceral brain-body information transfer. Neuroimage. 2009 Sep; 47 (3) :787-94. PubMed PMID:19446643.
- Canli T, Qiu M, Omura K, Congdon E, Haas BW, Amin Z, Herrmann MJ, Constable RT, Lesch KP. Neural correlates of epigenesis. Proc Natl Acad Sci U S A. 2006 Oct 24; 103 (43) :16033-8. PubMed PMID:17032778; PubMed Central PMCID: PMC1592642.
- Cao L, Liu X, Lin EJ, Wang C, Choi EY, Riban V, Lin B, During MJ. Environmental and genetic activation of a brain-adipocyte BDNF/leptin axis causes cancer remission and inhibition. Cell. 2010 Jul 9; 142 (1) :52-64. PubMed PMID:20603014.
- Carnethon MR. Physical Activity and Cardiovascular Disease: How Much is Enough?. Am J Lifestyle Med. 2009 Jul; 3 (1 Suppl) :44S-49S. PubMed PMID:20419076; PubMed Central PMCID: PMC2857374.
- Casey KL. Forebrain mechanisms of nociception and pain: analysis through imaging. Proc Natl Acad Sci U S A. 1999 Jul 6; 96 (14) :7668-74. PubMed PMID:10393878; PubMed Central PMCID: PMC33599.
- Cerqueira JJ, Almeida OF, Sousa N. The stressed prefrontal cortex Left? Right!. Brain Behav Immun. 2008 Jul; 22 (5) :630-8. PubMed PMID:18281193.
- Chen MJ, Yang WS, Yang JH, Hsiao CK, Yang YS, Ho HN. Low sex hormone-binding globulin is associated with low high-density

lipoprotein cholesterol and metabolic syndrome in women with PCOS. Hum Reprod. 2006 Sep; 21 (9) :2266-71. PubMed PMID:16757555.

- Chestnut, J.L. 2003. The 14 Foundational Premises for the Scientific and Philosophical Validation of the Chiropractic Wellness Paradigm. The Wellness Practice – Global Self Health Corp. Victoria, BC., Canada.
- Chestnut, J.L. 2004. The Innate Diet & Natural Hygiene. The Wellness Practice – Global Self Health Corp. Victoria, BC., Canada.
- Chestnut, J.L. 2005. Innate Physical Fitness & Spinal Hygiene. The Wellness Practice – Global Self Health Corp. Victoria, BC., Canada.
- Chestnut, J.L. 2005. The Innate State of Mind & Emotional Hygiene. The Wellness Practice – Global Self Health Corp. Victoria, BC., Canada.
- Chestnut, J.L. The Stroke Issue: Paucity of Valid Data, Plethora of Unsubstantiated Conjecture. J Manipulative Physiol Ther. June 2004 27 (5) :368-372
- Child et al. The impact of chiropractic care on established cardiac risk factors: A case study. The Journal of Chiropractic Research and Clinical Investigation
- Choobineh A, Lahmi M, Hosseini M, Shahnavaz H, Jazani RK. Workstation design in carpet hand-weaving operation: guidelines for prevention of musculoskeletal disorders. Int J Occup Saf Ergon. 2004; 10 (4) :411-24. PubMed PMID:15598364.
- Chopra, D. 1991, Perfect Health: the complete mind/body guide. Random House, Inc. New York, NY.
- Chrousos GP, Torpy DJ, Gold PW. Interactions between the hypothalamic-pituitary-adrenal axis and the female reproductive system: clinical implications. Ann Intern Med. 1998 Aug 1; 129 (3) :229-40. PubMed PMID:9696732.
- Cohen S, Tyrrell DA, Smith AP. Psychological stress and susceptibility to the common cold. N Engl J Med. 1991 Aug 29; 325 (9) :606-12. PubMed PMID:1713648.
- Collins A, Hill LE, Chandramohan Y, Whitcomb D, Droste SK, Reul JM. Exercise improves cognitive responses to psychological stress through enhancement of epigenetic mechanisms and gene expression in the

dentate gyrus. PLoS One. 2009; 4 (1) :e4330. PubMed PMID:19180197; PubMed Central PMCID: PMC2628725.

- Collins JJ, Baase CM, Sharda CE, et al. The assessment of chronic health conditions on work performance, absence, and total economic impact for employers. Journal of Occupational and Environmental Medicine. 2005;47:547-557.
- Cordain L, Miller JB, Eaton SB, Mann N, Holt SH, Speth JD. Plant-animal subsistence ratios and macronutrient energy estimations in worldwide hunter-gatherer diets. Am J Clin Nutr. 2000 Mar; 71 (3) :682-92. PubMed PMID:10702160.
- Cordain, Loren Ph.D. The Paleo Diet. John Wiley & Sons, Inc. New York 2002
- Cordain L, Gotshall RW, Eaton SB, Eaton SB 3rd. Physical activity, energy expenditure and fitness: an evolutionary perspective. Int J Sports Med. 1998 Jul; 19 (5) :328-35. PubMed PMID:9721056.
- Cordain L, Eaton SB, Sebastian A, Mann N, Lindeberg S, Watkins BA, O'Keefe JH, Brand-Miller J. Origins and evolution of the Western diet: health implications for the 21st century. Am J Clin Nutr. 2005 Feb; 81 (2) :341-54. PubMed PMID:15699220.
- Corrado E, Novo S. Evaluation of C-reactive protein in primary and secondary prevention. J Investig Med. 2007 Dec; 55 (8) :430-8. PubMed PMID:18163969.
- Covic M, Karaca E, Lie DC. Epigenetic regulation of neurogenesis in the adult hippocampus. Heredity. 2010 Jul; 105 (1) :122-34. PubMed PMID:20332807.
- Craig AD. Interoception: the sense of the physiological condition of the body. Curr Opin Neurobiol. 2003 Aug; 13 (4) :500-5. PubMed PMID:12965300.
- Craig AD. How do you feel? Interoception: the sense of the physiological condition of the body. Nat Rev Neurosci. 2002 Aug; 3 (8) :655-66. PubMed PMID:12154366.
- Crandall C, Palla S, Reboussin B, Hu P, Barrett-Connor E, Reuben D, Greendale G. Cross-sectional association between markers of inflammation and serum sex steroid levels in the postmenopausal

estrogen/progestin interventions trial. J Womens Health (Larchmt). 2006 Jan-Feb; 15 (1) :14-23. PubMed PMID:16417414.

- Curr Atheroscler Rep. 2001 Mar;3(2):174-9 Reviewed by Dr. J. Mercola www.mercola.com
- Davis, Devra. 2007. The Secret History of the War on Cancer. Basic Books. New York, NY.
- Davis JI, Senghas A, Brandt F, Ochsner KN. The effects of BOTOX injections on emotional experience. Emotion. 2010 Jun; 10 (3) :433-40. PubMed PMID:20515231; PubMed Central PMCID: PMC2880828.
- Davis-Floyd R. The technocratic, humanistic, and holistic paradigms of childbirth. Int J Gynaecol Obstet. 2001 Nov; 75 Suppl 1:S5-S23. PubMed PMID:11742639.
- De Bacquer D, De Backer G, Ostör E, Simon J, Pyörälä K, EUROASPIRE I Study Group. Predictive value of classical risk factors and their control in coronary patients: a follow-up of the EUROASPIRE I cohort. Eur J Cardiovasc Prev Rehabil. 2003 Aug; 10 (4) :289-95. PubMed PMID:14555885.
- De Meersman RE, Stein PK. Vagal modulation and aging. Biol Psychol. 2007 Feb; 74 (2) :165-73. PubMed PMID:17045727.
- Devilbiss DM, Page ME, Waterhouse BD. Locus ceruleus regulates sensory encoding by neurons and networks in waking animals. J Neurosci. 2006 Sep 27; 26 (39) :9860-72. PubMed PMID:17005850.
- DiPietro L, Dziura J, Yeckel CW, Neufer PD. Exercise and improved insulin sensitivity in older women: evidence of the enduring benefits of higher intensity training. J Appl Physiol. 2006 Jan; 100 (1) :142-9. PubMed PMID:16141382.
- Diamanti-Kandarakis E, Katsikis I, Piperi C, Alexandraki K, Panidis D. Effect of long-term orlistat treatment on serum levels of advanced glycation end-products in women with polycystic ovary syndrome. Clin Endocrinol (Oxf). 2007 Jan; 66 (1) :103-9. PubMed PMID:17201808.
- Doidge, Norman. 2007. The Brain That Changes Itself. Penguin Press. New York, NY.
- Douglas CC, Gower BA, Darnell BE, Ovalle F, Oster RA, Azziz R. Role

of diet in the treatment of polycystic ovary syndrome. Fertil Steril. 2006 Mar; 85 (3) :679-88. PubMed PMID:16500338.

- Dowd JB, Simanek AM, Aiello AE. Socio-economic status, cortisol and allostatic load: a review of the literature. Int J Epidemiol. 2009 Oct; 38 (5) :1297-309. PubMed PMID:19720725; PubMed Central PMCID: PMC2755130.
- Dudley R. Limits to human locomotor performance: phylogenetic origins and comparative perspectives. J Exp Biol. 2001 Sep; 204 (Pt 18) :3235-40. PubMed PMID:11581339.

- Eaton, Boyd M.D., Shostak, Marjorie., and Konner, Melvin M.D. Ph.D. The Paleolithic Prescription Harper and Row 1988
- Eaton SB, Konner M, Shostak M. Stone agers in the fast lane: chronic degenerative diseases in evolutionary perspective. Am J Med. 1988 Apr; 84 (4) :739-49. PubMed PMID:3135745.
- Eaton SB, Konner M. Paleolithic nutrition A consideration of its nature and current implications. N Engl J Med. 1985 Jan 31; 312 (5) :283-9. PubMed PMID:2981409.
- Eaton SB, Eaton SB 3rd, Konner MJ. Paleolithic nutrition revisited: a twelve-year retrospective on its nature and implications. Eur J Clin Nutr. 1997 Apr; 51 (4) :207-16. PubMed PMID:9104571.
- Eaton SB, Eaton SB. An evolutionary perspective on human physical activity: implications for health. Comp Biochem Physiol A Mol Integr Physiol. 2003 Sep; 136 (1) :153-9. PubMed PMID:14527637.
- Eaton SB, Strassman BI, Nesse RM, Neel JV, Ewald PW, Williams GC, Weder AB, Eaton SB 3rd, Lindeberg S, Konner MJ, Mysterud I, Cordain L. Evolutionary health promotion. Prev Med. 2002 Feb; 34 (2) :109-18. PubMed PMID:11817903.
- Eaton SB, Cordain L, Eaton SB. An evolutionary foundation for health promotion. World Rev Nutr Diet. 2001; 90:5-12. PubMed PMID:11545045.
- Eaton SB, Cordain L, Lindeberg S. Evolutionary health promotion: a consideration of common counterarguments. Prev Med. 2002 Feb; 34 (2) :119-23. PubMed PMID:11817904.

- Elenkov IJ, Wilder RL, Chrousos GP, Vizi ES. The sympathetic nerve--an integrative interface between two supersystems: the brain and the immune system. Pharmacol Rev. 2000 Dec; 52 (4) :595-638. PubMed PMID:11121511.
- Epel ES. Psychological and metabolic stress: a recipe for accelerated cellular aging?. Hormones (Athens). 2009 Jan-Mar; 8 (1) :7-22. PubMed PMID:19269917.
- Epel ES, McEwen B, Seeman T, Matthews K, Castellazzo G, Brownell KD, Bell J, Ickovics JR. Stress and body shape: stress-induced cortisol secretion is consistently greater among women with central fat. Psychosom Med. 2000 Sep-Oct; 62 (5) :623-32. PubMed PMID:11020091.
- Epel ES, Blackburn EH, Lin J, Dhabhar FS, Adler NE, Morrow JD, Cawthon RM. Accelerated telomere shortening in response to life stress. Proc Natl Acad Sci U S A. 2004 Dec 7; 101 (49) :17312-5. PubMed PMID:15574496; PubMed Central PMCID: PMC534658.
- Esch T, Stefano GB, Fricchione GL, Benson H. The role of stress in neurodegenerative diseases and mental disorders. Neuro Endocrinol Lett. 2002 Jun; 23 (3) :199-208. PubMed PMID:12080279.
- Esch T, Stefano GB, Fricchione GL, Benson H. Stress in cardiovascular diseases. Med Sci Monit. 2002 May; 8 (5) :RA93-RA101. PubMed PMID:12011786.
- Esch T, Fricchione GL, Stefano GB. The therapeutic use of the relaxation response in stress-related diseases. Med Sci Monit. 2003 Feb; 9 (2) :RA23-34. PubMed PMID:12601303.
- Expert Panel on Detection, Evaluation, and Treatment of High Blood Cholesterol in Adults. Executive Summary of The Third Report of The National Cholesterol Education Program (NCEP) Expert Panel on Detection, Evaluation, And Treatment of High Blood Cholesterol In Adults (Adult Treatment Panel III). JAMA. 2001 May 16; 285 (19) :2486-97. PubMed PMID:11368702.
- FDA Announces Qualified Health Claims for Omega-3 Fatty Acids September 8, 2004
- Fenoglio KA, Chen Y, Baram TZ. Neuroplasticity of the hypothalamic-pituitary-adrenal axis early in life requires recurrent recruitment of stress-regulating brain regions. J Neurosci. 2006 Mar 1; 26 (9) :2434-42.

PubMed PMID:16510721; PubMed Central PMCID: PMC2408688.

- Fletcher RH, Fairfield KM. Vitamins for chronic disease prevention in adults: clinical applications. JAMA. 2002 Jun 19; 287 (23) :3127-9. PubMed PMID:12069676.
- Fogarty AW, Glancy C, Jones S, Lewis SA, McKeever TM, Britton JR. A prospective study of weight change and systemic inflammation over 9 y. Am J Clin Nutr. 2008 Jan; 87 (1) :30-5. PubMed PMID:18175734.
- Ford ES, Bergmann MM, Kröger J, Schienkiewitz A, Weikert C, Boeing H. Healthy living is the best revenge: findings from the European Prospective Investigation Into Cancer and Nutrition-Potsdam study. Arch Intern Med. 2009 Aug 10; 169 (15) :1355-62. PubMed PMID:19667296.
- Franceschi, S. et al. Food groups and risk of colorectal cancer in Italy. Int. J. Cancer 1997 72:56-61.
- Frattaroli J, Weidner G, Merritt-Worden TA, Frenda S, Ornish D. Angina pectoris and atherosclerotic risk factors in the multisite cardiac lifestyle intervention program. Am J Cardiol. 2008 Apr 1; 101 (7) :911-8. PubMed PMID:18359307.
- Freburger JK, Holmes GM, Agans RP, Jackman AM, Darter JD, Wallace AS, Castel LD, Kalsbeek WD, Carey TS. The rising prevalence of chronic low back pain. Arch Intern Med. 2009 Feb 9; 169 (3) :251-8. PubMed PMID:19204216.
- Frost H, Lamb SE, Klaber Moffett JA, Fairbank JC, Moser JS. A fitness programme for patients with chronic low back pain: 2-year follow-up of a randomised controlled trial. Pain. 1998 Apr; 75 (2-3) :273-9. PubMed PMID:9583763.
- Furman EF, Gallo FP. 2000. The Neurophysics of Human Behavior. CRC Press LLC. New York, NY
- Galambos SA, Terry PC, Moyle GM, Locke SA, Lane AM. Psychological predictors of injury among elite athletes. Br J Sports Med. 2005 Jun; 39 (6) :351-4; discussion 351-4. PubMed PMID:15911606; PubMed Central PMCID: PMC1725228.
- Gann PH, Hennekens CH, Ma J, Longcope C, Stampfer MJ. Prospective study of sex hormone levels and risk of prostate cancer. J Natl Cancer

Inst. 1996 Aug 21; 88 (16) :1118-26. PubMed PMID:8757191.

- Geronimus AT, Hicken M, Keene D, Bound J. "Weathering" and age patterns of allostatic load scores among blacks and whites in the United States. Am J Public Health. 2006 May; 96 (5) :826-33. PubMed PMID:16380565; PubMed Central PMCID: PMC1470581.

- Ghadirian P, Narod S, Fafard E, Costa M, Robidoux A, Nkondjock A. Breast cancer risk in relation to the joint effect of BRCA mutations and diet diversity. Breast Cancer Res Treat. 2009 Sep; 117 (2) :417-22. PubMed PMID:19165595.

- Gibson GR, Beatty ER, Wang X, Cummings JH. Selective stimulation of bifidobacteria in the human colon by oligofructose and inulin. Gastroenterology. 1995 Apr; 108 (4) :975-82. PubMed PMID:7698613.

- Giese-Davis J, Conrad A, Nouriani B, Spiegel D. Exploring emotion-regulation and autonomic physiology in metastatic breast cancer patients: Repression, suppression, and restraint of hostility. Pers Individ Dif. 2008 Jan; 44 (1) :226-237. PubMed PMID:18461119; PubMed Central PMCID: PMC2836882.

- Gilbert MD. Weaving medicine back together: mind-body medicine in the twenty-first century. J Altern Complement Med. 2003 Aug; 9 (4) :563-70. PubMed PMID:14499032.

- Gimse R, Björgen IA, Tjell C, Tyssedal JS, Bø K. Reduced cognitive functions in a group of whiplash patients with demonstrated disturbances in the posture control system. J Clin Exp Neuropsychol. 1997 Dec; 19 (6) :838-49. PubMed PMID:9524878.

- Gluckman, Peter and Hanson, Mark. 2006. Mismatch: Why our world no longer fits our bodies. Oxford University Press.

- Goff et al. The effects of chiropractic adjustment on frontalis EMG potentials, spinal ranges of motion and anxiety level. J. of Chiro Res and Clin Investigation 1991

- González AS, Guerrero DB, Soto MB, Díaz SP, Martinez-Olmos M, Vidal O. Metabolic syndrome, insulin resistance and the inflammation markers C-reactive protein and ferritin. Eur J Clin Nutr. 2006 Jun; 60 (6) :802-9. PubMed PMID:16493453.

- Goodpaster BH, Delany JP, Otto AD, Kuller L, Vockley J, South-Paul

JE, Thomas SB, Brown J, McTigue K, Hames KC, Lang W, Jakicic JM. Effects of diet and physical activity interventions on weight loss and cardiometabolic risk factors in severely obese adults: a randomized trial. JAMA. 2010 Oct 27; 304 (16) :1795-802. PubMed PMID:20935337.

- Gosselin G, Rassoulian H, Brown I. Effects of neck extensor muscles fatigue on balance. Clin Biomech (Bristol, Avon). 2004 Jun; 19 (5) :473-9. PubMed PMID:15182982.
- Greider, Katharine. 2003. The Big Fix: How the Pharmaceutical Industry Rips Off American Consumers. Public Affairs. New York, NY.
- Griegel-Morris P, Larson K, Mueller-Klaus K, Oatis CA. Incidence of common postural abnormalities in the cervical, shoulder, and thoracic regions and their association with pain in two age groups of healthy subjects. Phys Ther. 1992 Jun; 72 (6) :425-31. PubMed PMID:1589462.
- Grounds MD, Radley HG, Gebski BL, Bogoyevitch MA, Shavlakadze T. Implications of cross-talk between tumour necrosis factor and insulin-like growth factor-1 signalling in skeletal muscle. Clin Exp Pharmacol Physiol. 2008 Jul; 35 (7) :846-51. PubMed PMID:18215180.
- Gruenewald TL, Seeman TE, Ryff CD, Karlamangla AS, Singer BH. Combinations of biomarkers predictive of later life mortality. Proc Natl Acad Sci U S A. 2006 Sep 19; 103 (38) :14158-63. PubMed PMID:16983099; PubMed Central PMCID: PMC1599928.
- Gu HF, Yang YM, Xu ZR. [Relationship between androgen levels and pathological changes of coronary atherosclerosis in elderly males]. Zhejiang Da Xue Xue Bao Yi Xue Ban. 2007 Jul; 36 (4) :382-5. PubMed PMID:17717831.
- Guyton. 1991. Textbook of Medical Physiology, Eighth Edition. W.B. Saunders Company. Philadelphia, PA.
- Haavik-Taylor, H. & Murphy, B. Cervical spine manipulation alters sensorimotor integration: A somatosensory evoked potential study. Clinical Neurophysiology 2007 118; 391-402
- Haby MM, Peat JK, Marks GB, Woolcock AJ, Leeder SR. Asthma in preschool children: prevalence and risk factors. Thorax. 2001 Aug; 56 (8) :589-95. PubMed PMID:11462059; PubMed Central PMCID: PMC1746115.

- Hall SA, Page ST, Travison TG, Montgomery RB, Link CL, McKinlay JB. Do statins affect androgen levels in men? Results from the Boston area community health survey. Cancer Epidemiol Biomarkers Prev. 2007 Aug; 16 (8) :1587-94. PubMed PMID:17684132.
- Hamburg NM, McMackin CJ, Huang AL, Shenouda SM, Widlansky ME, Schulz E, Gokce N, Ruderman NB, Keaney JF Jr, Vita JA. Physical inactivity rapidly induces insulin resistance and microvascular dysfunction in healthy volunteers. Arterioscler Thromb Vasc Biol. 2007 Dec; 27 (12) :2650-6. PubMed PMID:17932315; PubMed Central PMCID: PMC2596308.
- Hamilton MJ, Milne BT, Walker RS, Burger O, Brown JH. The complex structure of hunter-gatherer social networks. Proc Biol Sci. 2007 Sep 7; 274 (1622) :2195-202. PubMed PMID:17609186; PubMed Central PMCID: PMC2706200.
- Hardy K, Pollard H. The organisation of the stress response, and its relevance to chiropractors: a commentary. Chiropr Osteopat. 2006 Oct 18; 14:25. PubMed PMID:17044942; PubMed Central PMCID: PMC1629015.
- Hardy MP, Sottas CM, Ge R, McKittrick CR, Tamashiro KL, McEwen BS, Haider SG, Markham CM, Blanchard RJ, Blanchard DC, Sakai RR. Trends of reproductive hormones in male rats during psychosocial stress: role of glucocorticoid metabolism in behavioral dominance. Biol Reprod. 2002 Dec; 67 (6) :1750-5. PubMed PMID:12444049.
- Hayek, Ph.D 9th International Conference on Spinal Manipulation Oct 5, 2002 Reported in Advance 23 (2) Foundation for Chiropractic Education and Research.
- Heath, Chip and Dan. 2010. Switch: How to Change Things When Change Is Hard. Random House. New York, NY
- Hildebrandt AL, Pilegaard H, Neufer PD. Differential transcriptional activation of select metabolic genes in response to variations in exercise intensity and duration. Am J Physiol Endocrinol Metab. 2003 Nov; 285 (5) :E1021-7. PubMed PMID:12902322.
- Hjerkinn EM, Sandvik L, Hjermann I, Arnesen H. Effect of diet intervention on long-term mortality in healthy middle-aged men with combined hyperlipidaemia. J Intern Med. 2004 Jan; 255 (1) :68-73.

PubMed PMID:14687240.

- Hoosmand, Hooshang, Chronic pain: reflex sympathetic dystrophy, prevention and management CRC Press 1993
- Holme I, Tonstad S, Sogaard AJ, Larsen PG, Haheim LL. Leisure time physical activity in middle age predicts the metabolic syndrome in old age: results of a 28-year follow-up of men in the Oslo study. BMC Public Health. 2007 Jul 12; 7:154. PubMed PMID:17625024; PubMed Central PMCID: PMC1947967.
- Houlihan et al "Body Burden: The Pollution in Newborns," Environmental Working Group, July 14, 2005.
- Hubley-Kozey CL, Vezina MJ. Differentiating temporal electromyographic waveforms between those with chronic low back pain and healthy controls. Clin Biomech (Bristol, Avon). 2002 Nov-Dec; 17 (9-10) :621-9. PubMed PMID:12446158.
- Hunter RG, McCarthy KJ, Milne TA, Pfaff DW, McEwen BS. Regulation of hippocampal H3 histone methylation by acute and chronic stress. Proc Natl Acad Sci U S A. 2009 Dec 8; 106 (49) :20912-7. PubMed PMID:19934035; PubMed Central PMCID: PMC2791599.
- Hwang JS, Wu TL, Chou SC, Ho C, Chang PY, Tsao KC, Huang JY, Sun CF, Wu JT. Development of multiple complications in type 2 diabetes is associated with the increase of multiple markers of chronic inflammation. J Clin Lab Anal. 2008; 22 (1) :6-13. PubMed PMID:18200579.
- Hyman MA, Ornish D, Roizen M. Lifestyle medicine: treating the causes of disease. Altern Ther Health Med. 2009 Nov-Dec; 15 (6) :12-4. PubMed PMID:19943572.
- Høstmark AT. [Physical activity and plasma lipids]. Tidsskr Nor Laegeforen. 1980 May 5; 100 (12B) :771-6. PubMed PMID:7404518.
- Imani F, Kehoe KE. Infection of human B lymphocytes with MMR vaccine induces IgE class switching. Clin Immunol. 2001 Sep; 100 (3) :355-61. PubMed PMID:11513549.
- Irigaray P, Newby JA, Clapp R, Hardell L, Howard V, Montagnier L, Epstein S, Belpomme D. Lifestyle-related factors and environmental agents causing cancer: an overview. Biomed Pharmacother. 2007 Dec; 61

(10) :640-58. PubMed PMID:18055160.

- Itoi E, Sinaki M. Effect of back-strengthening exercise on posture in healthy women 49 to 65 years of age. Mayo Clin Proc. 1994 Nov; 69 (11) :1054-9. PubMed PMID:7967758.
- Itzkowitz SH, Yio X. Inflammation and cancer IV Colorectal cancer in inflammatory bowel disease: the role of inflammation. Am J Physiol Gastrointest Liver Physiol. 2004 Jul; 287 (1) :G7-17. PubMed PMID:15194558.
- Jenkins DJ, Kendall CW, Marchie A, Jenkins AL, Connelly PW, Jones PJ, Vuksan V. The Garden of Eden--plant based diets, the genetic drive to conserve cholesterol and its implications for heart disease in the 21st century. Comp Biochem Physiol A Mol Integr Physiol. 2003 Sep; 136 (1) :141-51. PubMed PMID:14527636.
- Jensen, E. Learning with the body in mind. 2000.
- Jensen, E. Brain-Based Learning. The Brain Store 1995 San Diego, CA USA
- Jensen, E. Brain-Based Learning: The new science of teaching and training. 2000.
- Johnson GM. The correlation between surface measurement of head and neck posture and the anatomic position of the upper cervical vertebrae. Spine (Phila Pa 1976). 1998 Apr 15; 23 (8) :921-7. PubMed PMID:9580960.
- Johnston-Brooks CH, Lewis MA, Evans GW, Whalen CK. Chronic stress and illness in children: the role of allostatic load. Psychosom Med. 1998 Sep-Oct; 60 (5) :597-603. PubMed PMID:9773764.
- Jones, David S., MD, Hofmann, Laurie, MPH. Quinn, Sheila. 2009. 21st century medicine: A New Model for Medical Education and Practice. The Institute for Functional Medicine.
- Jump DB. Dietary polyunsaturated fatty acids and regulation of gene transcription. Curr Opin Lipidol. 2002 Apr; 13 (2) :155-64. PubMed PMID:11891418.
- Jönsson T, Granfeldt Y, Ahrén B, Branell UC, Pålsson G, Hansson A, Söderström M, Lindeberg S. Beneficial effects of a Paleolithic diet on cardiovascular risk factors in type 2 diabetes: a randomized cross-

over pilot study. Cardiovasc Diabetol. 2009 Jul 16; 8:35. PubMed PMID:19604407; PubMed Central PMCID: PMC2724493.

- Kado DM, Huang MH, Karlamangla AS, Barrett-Connor E, Greendale GA. Hyperkyphotic posture predicts mortality in older community-dwelling men and women: a prospective study. J Am Geriatr Soc. 2004 Oct; 52 (10) :1662-7. PubMed PMID:15450042.

- Karim R, Hodis HN, Stanczyk FZ, Lobo RA, Mack WJ. Relationship between serum levels of sex hormones and progression of subclinical atherosclerosis in postmenopausal women. J Clin Endocrinol Metab. 2008 Jan; 93 (1) :131-8. PubMed PMID:17925335; PubMed Central PMCID: PMC2190735.

- Karlamangla AS, Singer BH, Seeman TE. Reduction in allostatic load in older adults is associated with lower all-cause mortality risk: MacArthur studies of successful aging. Psychosom Med. 2006 May-Jun; 68 (3) :500-7. PubMed PMID:16738085.

- Keller TS, Colloca CJ. Mechanical force spinal manipulation increases trunk muscle strength assessed by electromyography: a comparative clinical trial. J Manipulative Physiol Ther. 2000 Nov-Dec; 23 (9) :585-95. PubMed PMID:11145798.

- Kendrick, Malcolm M.D. Why The Cholesterol-Heart Disease Theory Is Wrong. Feb. 14, 2003 Redflagsweekly.com

- Kessler, A. 2006. The End of Medicine. Harper Collins Publishers. New York, NY.

- Kilo CM, Larson EB. Exploring the harmful effects of health care. JAMA. 2009 Jul 1; 302 (1) :89-91. PubMed PMID:19567446.

- Klein N, Fröhlich F, Krief S. Geophagy: soil consumption enhances the bioactivities of plants eaten by chimpanzees. Naturwissenschaften. 2008 Apr; 95 (4) :325-31. PubMed PMID:18188538.

- Kogler A, Lindfors J, Odkvist LM, Ledin T. Postural stability using different neck positions in normal subjects and patients with neck trauma. Acta Otolaryngol. 2000 Mar; 120 (2) :151-5. PubMed PMID:11603761.

- Korte SM, Prins J, Vinkers CH, Olivier B. On the origin of allostasis and stress-induced pathology in farm animals: celebrating Darwin's legacy.

Vet J. 2009 Dec; 182 (3) :378-83. PubMed PMID:19747860.

- Kotrschal A, Ilmonen P, Penn DJ. Stress impacts telomere dynamics. Biol Lett. 2007 Apr 22; 3 (2) :128-30. PubMed PMID:17264051; PubMed Central PMCID: PMC2375929.
- Krieger DR, Landsberg L. Mechanisms in obesity-related hypertension: role of insulin and catecholamines. Am J Hypertens. 1988 Jan; 1 (1) :84-90. PubMed PMID:3285861.
- Kroemer and Grandjean. "Mental Activity" and "Fatigue". Fitting the task to the Human: A textbook of Occupational Ergonomics. 1997
- Kuhn, Thomas S. 1962. The Structure of Scientific Revolutions. University of Chicago Press.
- Kuukkanen T, Mälkiä E. Muscular performance after a 3 month progressive physical exercise program and 9 month follow-up in subjects with low back pain A controlled study. Scand J Med Sci Sports. 1996 Apr; 6 (2) :112-21. PubMed PMID:8809928.
- Kuukkanen TM, Mälkiä EA. An experimental controlled study on postural sway and therapeutic exercise in subjects with low back pain. Clin Rehabil. 2000 Apr; 14 (2) :192-202. PubMed PMID:10763797.
- Lada AT, Rudel LL, St Clair RW. Effects of LDL enriched with different dietary fatty acids on cholesteryl ester accumulation and turnover in THP-1 macrophages. J Lipid Res. 2003 Apr; 44 (4) :770-9. PubMed PMID:12562836.
- Landsberg L. Insulin-mediated sympathetic stimulation: role in the pathogenesis of obesity-related hypertension (or, how insulin affects blood pressure, and why). J Hypertens. 2001 Mar; 19 (3 Pt 2) :523-8. PubMed PMID:11327624.
- Latendresse G. The interaction between chronic stress and pregnancy: preterm birth from a biobehavioral perspective. J Midwifery Womens Health. 2009 Jan-Feb; 54 (1) :8-17. PubMed PMID:19114234; PubMed Central PMCID: PMC2651684.
- Lauro and Mouch. Chiropractic effects on athletic ability J. of Chiro Res and Clin Invest 1991
- Lee H, Nicholson LL, Adams RD. Cervical range of motion associations

with subclinical neck pain. Spine (Phila Pa 1976). 2004 Jan 1; 29 (1) :33-40. PubMed PMID:14699273.

- Lee WY, Okeson JP, Lindroth J. The relationship between forward head posture and temporomandibular disorders. J Orofac Pain. 1995 Spring; 9 (2) :161-7. PubMed PMID:7488986.
- Leinonen V, Kankaanpää M, Luukkonen M, Kansanen M, Hänninen O, Airaksinen O, Taimela S. Lumbar paraspinal muscle function, perception of lumbar position, and postural control in disc herniation-related back pain. Spine (Phila Pa 1976). 2003 Apr 15; 28 (8) :842-8. PubMed PMID:12698130.
- Lennon et al. Postural and respiratory modulation of autonomic function, pain, and health. Am J Pain Manage 1994 (4) 36-39
- Li S, Zhao JH, Luan J, Ekelund U, Luben RN, Khaw KT, Wareham NJ, Loos RJ. Physical activity attenuates the genetic predisposition to obesity in 20,000 men and women from EPIC-Norfolk prospective population study. PLoS Med. 2010 Aug 31; 7 (8) PubMed PMID:20824172; PubMed Central PMCID: PMC2930873.
- Lianov L, Johnson M. Physician competencies for prescribing lifestyle medicine. JAMA. 2010 Jul 14; 304 (2) :202-3. PubMed PMID:20628134.
- Liebenson, Craig. Rehabilitation of the Spine: A Practitioner's Manual 1996 William & Wilkins Pennsylvania U.S.A.
- Lindberg G, Lindblad U, Löw-Larsen B, Merlo J, Melander A, Råstam L. Use of calcium channel blockers as antihypertensives in relation to mortality and cancer incidence: a population-based observational study. Pharmacoepidemiol Drug Saf. 2002 Sep; 11 (6) :493-7. PubMed PMID:12426934.
- Lindeberg S, Söderberg S, Ahrén B, Olsson T. Large differences in serum leptin levels between nonwesternized and westernized populations: the Kitava study. J Intern Med. 2001 Jun; 249 (6) :553-8. PubMed PMID:11422662.
- Lipton, BH. 2005. The Biology of Belief: unleashing the power of consciousness matter and miracles. Mountain of Love/Elite Books. Santa Rosa, CA.
- Lipton HL. Home is where the health is: advancing team-based care in

chronic disease management. Arch Intern Med. 2009 Nov 23; 169 (21) :1945-8. PubMed PMID:19933953.

- Logan JG, Barksdale DJ. Allostasis and allostatic load: expanding the discourse on stress and cardiovascular disease. J Clin Nurs. 2008 Apr; 17 (7B) :201-8. PubMed PMID:18578796.
- Lorig KR, Laurent DD, Deyo RA, Marnell ME, Minor MA, Ritter PL. Can a Back Pain E-mail Discussion Group improve health status and lower health care costs?: A randomized study. Arch Intern Med. 2002 Apr 8; 162 (7) :792-6. PubMed PMID:11926853.
- Low YL, Dunning AM, Dowsett M, Luben RN, Khaw KT, Wareham NJ, Bingham SA. Implications of gene-environment interaction in studies of gene variants in breast cancer: an example of dietary isoflavones and the D356N polymorphism in the sex hormone-binding globulin gene. Cancer Res. 2006 Sep 15; 66 (18) :8980-3. PubMed PMID:16982738.
- Lowery, G. Three-dimensional screw divergence and sagittal balance: a personal philosophy relative to cervical biomechanics. Spine: State of the Art Reviews 1996; 10:342-56
- Luoto S, Taimela S, Hurri H, Alaranta H. Mechanisms explaining the association between low back trouble and deficits in information processing A controlled study with follow-up. Spine (Phila Pa 1976). 1999 Feb 1; 24 (3) :255-61. PubMed PMID:10025020.
- Luoto S, Aalto H, Taimela S, Hurri H, Pyykkö I, Alaranta H. One-footed and externally disturbed two-footed postural control in patients with chronic low back pain and healthy control subjects A controlled study with follow-up. Spine (Phila Pa 1976). 1998 Oct 1; 23 (19) :2081-9; discussion 2089-90. PubMed PMID:9794052.
- MacKelvie KJ, Khan KM, Petit MA, Janssen PA, McKay HA. A school-based exercise intervention elicits substantial bone health benefits: a 2-year randomized controlled trial in girls. Pediatrics. 2003 Dec; 112 (6 Pt 1) :e447. PubMed PMID:14654643.
- Magno Zito J et.al. Trends in Prescribing Psychotropic Medications to Preschoolers. JAMA . 2000;283:1025-1030.
- Maliqueo M, Bacallao K, Quezada S, Clementi M, Gabler F, Johnson MC, Vega M. Sex hormone-binding globulin expression in the endometria of women with polycystic ovary syndrome. Fertil Steril. 2007

Feb; 87 (2) :321-8. PubMed PMID:17097651.

- Mann SJ. The mind/body link in essential hypertension: time for a new paradigm. Altern Ther Health Med. 2000 Mar; 6 (2) :39-45. PubMed PMID:10710802.
- Mann WA. [Impact of lifestyle changes on hypertension and diabetes]. MMW Fortschr Med. 2004 May 27; 146 (22) :28-30. PubMed PMID:15373105.
- Mann, NJ. 2004 Paleolithic Nutrition: What can we learn from the past? Asia Pac J Clin Nutr : 13 (Suppl): S17
- Manson JE, Skerrett PJ, Greenland P, VanItallie TB. The escalating pandemics of obesity and sedentary lifestyle A call to action for clinicians. Arch Intern Med. 2004 Feb 9; 164 (3) :249-58. PubMed PMID:14769621.
- Manta S, Dong J, Debonnel G, Blier P. Enhancement of the function of rat serotonin and norepinephrine neurons by sustained vagus nerve stimulation. J Psychiatry Neurosci. 2009 Jul; 34 (4) :272-80. PubMed PMID:19568478; PubMed Central PMCID: PMC2702444.
- Marshall DA, Walizer E, Vernalis MN. Optimal healing environments for chronic cardiovascular disease. J Altern Complement Med. 2004; 10 Suppl 1:S147-55. PubMed PMID:15630832.
- Martin CK, Church TS, Thompson AM, Earnest CP, Blair SN. Exercise dose and quality of life: a randomized controlled trial. Arch Intern Med. 2009 Feb 9; 169 (3) :269-78. PubMed PMID:19204218; PubMed Central PMCID: PMC2745102.
- Martinez-Lavin M, Vargas A. Complex adaptive systems allostasis in fibromyalgia. Rheum Dis Clin North Am. 2009 May; 35 (2) :285-98. PubMed PMID:19647143.
- Mathison R, Davison JS, Befus AD. Neuroendocrine regulation of inflammation and tissue repair by submandibular gland factors. Immunol Today. 1994 Nov; 15 (11) :527-32. PubMed PMID:7802923.
- Mathison RD, Davison JS, Befus AD. A peptide from the submandibular glands modulates inflammatory responses. Int Arch Allergy Immunol. 1997 May-Jul; 113 (1-3) :337-8. PubMed PMID:9130570.

- McAnalley, B. Ph.D. & Vennum, E. RAC Glycoscience: State of the Science Review. Glycoscience and Nutrition 2001: 2 (14)
- McDermott, Ian & O'Connor Joseph 'NLP (Neuro-Linguistic-Programming) and Health' Thorsons 1996
- McEwen BS. The neurobiology of stress: from serendipity to clinical relevance. Brain Res. 2000 Dec 15; 886 (1-2) :172-189. PubMed PMID:11119695.
- McEwen BS. Physiology and neurobiology of stress and adaptation: central role of the brain. Physiol Rev. 2007 Jul; 87 (3) :873-904. PubMed PMID:17615391.
- McEwen BS. Plasticity of the hippocampus: adaptation to chronic stress and allostatic load. Ann N Y Acad Sci. 2001 Mar; 933:265-77. PubMed PMID:12000027.
- McEwen BS. Sex, stress and the hippocampus: allostasis, allostatic load and the aging process. Neurobiol Aging. 2002 Sep-Oct; 23 (5) :921-39. PubMed PMID:12392796.
- McEwen BS. Central effects of stress hormones in health and disease: Understanding the protective and damaging effects of stress and stress mediators. Eur J Pharmacol. 2008 Apr 7; 583 (2-3) :174-85. PubMed PMID:18282566; PubMed Central PMCID: PMC2474765.
- McEwen BS, Wingfield JC. What is in a name? Integrating homeostasis, allostasis and stress. Horm Behav. 2010 Feb; 57 (2) :105-11. PubMed PMID:19786032; PubMed Central PMCID: PMC2815096.
- McEwen BS, Milner TA. Hippocampal formation: shedding light on the influence of sex and stress on the brain. Brain Res Rev. 2007 Oct; 55 (2) :343-55. PubMed PMID:17395265; PubMed Central PMCID: PMC2101766.
- McEwen BS. Stressed or stressed out: what is the difference?. J Psychiatry Neurosci. 2005 Sep; 30 (5) :315-8. PubMed PMID:16151535; PubMed Central PMCID: PMC1197275.
- McEwen BS. Commentary: the ever-changing brain. Neuropsychopharmacology. 2001 Dec; 25 (6) :797-8. PubMed PMID:11750173.

- McEwen BS. Allostasis and allostatic load: implications for neuropsychopharmacology. Neuropsychopharmacology. 2000 Feb; 22 (2) :108-24. PubMed PMID:10649824.
- McEwen BS. Allostasis, allostatic load, and the aging nervous system: role of excitatory amino acids and excitotoxicity. Neurochem Res. 2000 Oct; 25 (9-10) :1219-31. PubMed PMID:11059796.
- McEwen BS, Stellar E. Stress and the individual Mechanisms leading to disease. Arch Intern Med. 1993 Sep 27; 153 (18) :2093-101. PubMed PMID:8379800.
- McGill, S. Stability: from biomechanical concept to chiropractic practice. JCCA 1999; 43 (2)
- McGregor et al. Immunological response to manipulation of the lumbar spine. ICSM Proceedings 1991. * Asymptomatic Subjects
- McKnight ME, DeBoer KF. Preliminary study of blood pressure changes in normotensive subjects undergoing chiropractic care. J Manipulative Physiol Ther. 1988 Aug; 11 (4) :261-6. PubMed PMID:3171413.
- McTaggart, Lynne. What Doctors Don't Tell You: The truth about the dangers of modern medicine. Avon Books New York, New York 1996.
- Meaney, Michael PhD Stress and Disease: Who Gets Sick: Who Stays Well Cortext Educational Seminars Fall, 2001
- Metcalfe KA, Finch A, Poll A, Horsman D, Kim-Sing C, Scott J, Royer R, Sun P, Narod SA. Breast cancer risks in women with a family history of breast or ovarian cancer who have tested negative for a BRCA1 or BRCA2 mutation. Br J Cancer. 2009 Jan 27; 100 (2) :421-5. PubMed PMID:19088722; PubMed Central PMCID: PMC2634722.
- Mientjes MI, Frank JS. Balance in chronic low back pain patients compared to healthy people under various conditions in upright standing. Clin Biomech (Bristol, Avon). 1999 Dec; 14 (10) :710-6. PubMed PMID:10545625.
- Miller et al. The effect of spinal manipulation and soft tissue massage on human endurance and cardiac and pulmonary physiology: A pilot study. J. of Sports Chiro and Rehab 2000
- Möltner A, Hölzl R. Interoception, body perception and awareness The

heritage of György Adám. Acta Biol Hung. 2002; 53 (4) :515-36. PubMed PMID:12501936.

- Müller SV, von Schweder AJ, Frank B, Dengler R, Münte TF, Johannes S. The effects of proprioceptive stimulation on cognitive processes in patients after traumatic brain injury. Arch Phys Med Rehabil. 2002 Jan; 83 (1) :115-21. PubMed PMID:11782841.
- Nagasawa A, Sakakibara T, Takahashi A. Roentgenographic findings of the cervical spine in tension-type headache. Headache. 1993 Feb; 33 (2) :90-5. PubMed PMID:8458729.
- Nance DM, Sanders VM. Autonomic innervation and regulation of the immune system (1987-2007). Brain Behav Immun. 2007 Aug; 21 (6) :736-45. PubMed PMID:17467231; PubMed Central PMCID: PMC1986730.
- Nansel D, Jansen R, Cremata E, Dhami MS, Holley D. Effects of cervical adjustments on lateral-flexion passive end-range asymmetry and on blood pressure, heart rate and plasma catecholamine levels. J Manipulative Physiol Ther. 1991 Oct; 14 (8) :450-6. PubMed PMID:1940682.
- Nansel DD, Cremata E, Carlson J, Szlazak M. Effect of unilateral spinal adjustments on goniometrically-assessed cervical lateral-flexion end-range asymmetries in otherwise asymptomatic subjects. J Manipulative Physiol Ther. 1989 Dec; 12 (6) :419-27. PubMed PMID:2486560.
- Nansel DD, Peneff A, Quitoriano J. Effectiveness of upper versus lower cervical adjustments with respect to the amelioration of passive rotational versus lateral-flexion end-range asymmetries in otherwise asymptomatic subjects. J Manipulative Physiol Ther. 1992 Feb; 15 (2) :99-105. PubMed PMID:1564415.
- Nash DT. Relationship of C-reactive protein, metabolic syndrome and diabetes mellitus: potential role of statins. J Natl Med Assoc. 2005 Dec; 97 (12) :1600-7. PubMed PMID:16396052; PubMed Central PMCID: PMC2640717.
- New York Times December 23, 2003 More Than One-Third of Those Born in 2000 Will Get Diabetes
- Niclis C, Del Pilar Díaz M, La Vecchia C. Breast cancer mortality trends and patterns in Córdoba, Argentina in the period 1986-2006. Eur J Cancer Prev. 2010 Mar; 19 (2) :94-9. PubMed PMID:20051872.

- Nijm J, Kristenson M, Olsson AG, Jonasson L. Impaired cortisol response to acute stressors in patients with coronary disease Implications for inflammatory activity. J Intern Med. 2007 Sep; 262 (3) :375-84. PubMed PMID:17697159.
- O'Dea K. Marked improvement in carbohydrate and lipid metabolism in diabetic Australian aborigines after temporary reversion to traditional lifestyle. Diabetes. 1984 Jun; 33 (6) :596-603. PubMed PMID:6373464.
- O'Keefe JH Jr, Cordain L. Cardiovascular disease resulting from a diet and lifestyle at odds with our Paleolithic genome: how to become a 21st-century hunter-gatherer. Mayo Clin Proc. 2004 Jan; 79 (1) :101-8. PubMed PMID:14708953.
- Obomsawin , Raymond. 2007. Historical and Scientific Perspectives on the health of Canada's First Peoples. March, 2007
- Onat A, Hergenç G, Karabulut A, Albayrak S, Can G, Kaya Z. Serum sex hormone-binding globulin, a determinant of cardiometabolic disorders independent of abdominal obesity and insulin resistance in elderly men and women. Metabolism. 2007 Oct; 56 (10) :1356-62. PubMed PMID:17884445.
- Ornish D, Weidner G, Fair WR, Marlin R, Pettengill EB, Raisin CJ, Dunn-Emke S, Crutchfield L, Jacobs FN, Barnard RJ, Aronson WJ, McCormac P, McKnight DJ, Fein JD, Dnistrian AM, Weinstein J, Ngo TH, Mendell NR, Carroll PR. Intensive lifestyle changes may affect the progression of prostate cancer. J Urol. 2005 Sep; 174 (3) :1065-9; discussion 1069-70. PubMed PMID:16094059.
- Ornish D, Magbanua MJ, Weidner G, Weinberg V, Kemp C, Green C, Mattie MD, Marlin R, Simko J, Shinohara K, Haqq CM, Carroll PR. Changes in prostate gene expression in men undergoing an intensive nutrition and lifestyle intervention. Proc Natl Acad Sci U S A. 2008 Jun 17; 105 (24) :8369-74. PubMed PMID:18559852; PubMed Central PMCID: PMC2430265.
- Ornish D, Scherwitz LW, Billings JH, Brown SE, Gould KL, Merritt TA, Sparler S, Armstrong WT, Ports TA, Kirkeeide RL, Hogeboom C, Brand RJ. Intensive lifestyle changes for reversal of coronary heart disease. JAMA. 1998 Dec 16; 280 (23) :2001-7. PubMed PMID:9863851.
- Ornish D, Lin J, Daubenmier J, Weidner G, Epel E, Kemp C, Magbanua

MJ, Marlin R, Yglecias L, Carroll PR, Blackburn EH. Increased telomerase activity and comprehensive lifestyle changes: a pilot study. Lancet Oncol. 2008 Nov; 9 (11) :1048-57. PubMed PMID:18799354.

- Ornish D. Reversing heart disease through diet, exercise, and stress management: an interview with Dean Ornish Interview by Elaine R Monsen. J Am Diet Assoc. 1991 Feb; 91 (2) :162-5. PubMed PMID:1991929.
- Ottaway CA. Role of the neuroendocrine system in cytokine pathways in inflammatory bowel disease. Aliment Pharmacol Ther. 1996; 10 Suppl 2:10-5. PubMed PMID:8899096.
- Paradies YC, Montoya MJ, Fullerton SM. Racialized genetics and the study of complex diseases: the thrifty genotype revisited. Perspect Biol Med. 2007 Spring; 50 (2) :203-27. PubMed PMID:17468539.
- Perzigian AJ. Osteoporotic bone loss in two prehistoric Indian populations. Am J Phys Anthropol. 1973 Jul; 39 (1) :87-95. PubMed PMID:4351578.
- Pikalov and Kharin. Use of spinal manipulative treatment as complementary therapy following surgery: A prospective match controlled outcome study Alternative Therapies 2000
- Pilegaard H, Ordway GA, Saltin B, Neufer PD. Transcriptional regulation of gene expression in human skeletal muscle during recovery from exercise. Am J Physiol Endocrinol Metab. 2000 Oct; 279 (4) :E806-14. PubMed PMID:11001762.
- Pischke CR, Scherwitz L, Weidner G, Ornish D. Long-term effects of lifestyle changes on well-being and cardiac variables among coronary heart disease patients. Health Psychol. 2008 Sep; 27 (5) :584-92. PubMed PMID:18823185.
- Pollack, Gerald H. 2001. Cells, Gels and the Engines of Life: A New, Unifying Approach to Cell Function. Ebner and Sons Publishers, Seattle, WA.
- Pollan, Michael. 2006. The Omnivore's Dilemma: A Natural History of Four Meals. The Penguin Press.
- Pollard and Ward. Strength change of quadriceps femoris following a single manipulation of the L3/L4 vertebral motion segment: A

preliminary investigation JNMS 1996

- Popovich DG, Jenkins DJ, Kendall CW, Dierenfeld ES, Carroll RW, Tariq N, Vidgen E. The western lowland gorilla diet has implications for the health of humans and other hominoids. J Nutr. 1997 Oct; 127 (10) :2000-5. PubMed PMID:9311957.
- Powell JP, Leonard JS. A nutritional program improved lipid profiles and weight in 28 chiropractic patients: a retrospective case series. J Chiropr Med. 2008 Sep; 7 (3) :94-100. PubMed PMID:19646370; PubMed Central PMCID: PMC2686396.
- Power, Michael. L. in Schulkin, Jay. (2004). Allostasis, Homeostasis, and the Costs of Physiological Adaptation. Cambridge University Press. Cambridge, U.K.
- Praet SF, Jonkers RA, Schep G, Stehouwer CD, Kuipers H, Keizer HA, van Loon LJ. Long-standing, insulin-treated type 2 diabetes patients with complications respond well to short-term resistance and interval exercise training. Eur J Endocrinol. 2008 Feb; 158 (2) :163-72. PubMed PMID:18230822.
- Radebold A, Cholewicki J, Polzhofer GK, Greene HS. Impaired postural control of the lumbar spine is associated with delayed muscle response times in patients with chronic idiopathic low back pain. Spine (Phila Pa 1976). 2001 Apr 1; 26 (7) :724-30. PubMed PMID:11295888.
- Radley JJ, Williams B, Sawchenko PE. Noradrenergic innervation of the dorsal medial prefrontal cortex modulates hypothalamo-pituitary-adrenal responses to acute emotional stress. J Neurosci. 2008 May 28; 28 (22) :5806-16. PubMed PMID:18509042; PubMed Central PMCID: PMC2796223.
- Ramberg, J. M.S. and McAnalley, B. Ph.D. Is saccharide supplementation necessary? Glycoscience and Nutrition 2002: 3 (3)
- Ramos BP, Arnsten AF. Adrenergic pharmacology and cognition: focus on the prefrontal cortex. Pharmacol Ther. 2007 Mar; 113 (3) :523-36. PubMed PMID:17303246; PubMed Central PMCID: PMC2151919.
- Rand KL. The return of science to education in clinical psychology: a reply to Snyder and Elliott. J Clin Psychol. 2005 Sep; 61 (9) :1185-90. PubMed PMID:15965945.

- Rannou F, Ouanes W, Boutron I, Lovisi B, Fayad F, Macé Y, Borderie D, Guerini H, Poiraudeau S, Revel M. High-sensitivity C-reactive protein in chronic low back pain with vertebral end-plate Modic signal changes. Arthritis Rheum. 2007 Oct 15; 57 (7) :1311-5. PubMed PMID:17907216.
- Rately, John. 2008. Spark: the revolutionary new science of exercise and the brain. New York, NY. Little, Brown and Company.
- Reiche EM, Morimoto HK, Nunes SM. Stress and depression-induced immune dysfunction: implications for the development and progression of cancer. Int Rev Psychiatry. 2005 Dec; 17 (6) :515-27. PubMed PMID:16401550.
- Ren K, Novikova SI, He F, Dubner R, Lidow MS. Neonatal local noxious insult affects gene expression in the spinal dorsal horn of adult rats. Mol Pain. 2005 Sep 22; 1:27. PubMed PMID:16179088; PubMed Central PMCID: PMC1242251.
- Reseland JE, Anderssen SA, Solvoll K, Hjermann I, Urdal P, Holme I, Drevon CA. Effect of long-term changes in diet and exercise on plasma leptin concentrations. Am J Clin Nutr. 2001 Feb; 73 (2) :240-5. PubMed PMID:11157319.
- Restak, R.M. (1979) The Brain: The last frontier.
- Rhoades and Pflanzer. 1989. Human Physiology. Saunders College Publishing. Philadelphia, PA.
- Rippe JM, Angelopoulos TJ, Rippe WF. Lifestyle Medicine and Health Care Reform. Am J Lifestyle Med. Nov/Dec 2009.
- Rippe JM, Angelopoulos TJ. Physical activity and health: the time for action is now. Am J Lifestyle Med. May/Jun 2010
- Rittweger J, Just K, Kautzsch K, Reeg P, Felsenberg D. Treatment of chronic lower back pain with lumbar extension and whole-body vibration exercise: a randomized controlled trial. Spine (Phila Pa 1976). 2002 Sep 1; 27 (17) :1829-34. PubMed PMID:12221343.
- Roberts CK, Barnard RJ. Effects of exercise and diet on chronic disease. J Appl Physiol. 2005 Jan; 98 (1) :3-30. PubMed PMID:15591300.
- Robinson MJ, Edwards SE, Iyengar S, Bymaster F, Clark M, Katon W. Depression and pain. Front Biosci. 2009 Jun 1; 14:5031-51. PubMed

PMID:19482603.

- Rogers AE. Methyl donors in the diet and responses to chemical carcinogens. Am J Clin Nutr. 1995 Mar; 61 (3 Suppl) :659S-665S. PubMed PMID:7879734.
- Romero LM, Dickens MJ, Cyr NE. The Reactive Scope Model - a new model integrating homeostasis, allostasis, and stress. Horm Behav. 2009 Mar; 55 (3) :375-89. PubMed PMID:19470371.
- Román O, Cuevas G, Badilla M, Valenzuela A, Cumsille F, Valverde L, Rodríguez N. [Morbidity and mortality of treated essential arterial hypertension in a 26 years follow up]. Rev Med Chil. 2002 Apr; 130 (4) :379-86. PubMed PMID:12090102.
- Ruff CB, Trinkaus E, Holliday T. Body mass and encephalization in Pleistocene HomoNature 387, 173 - 176 (08 May 1997)
- Ruiz JR, Sui X, Lobelo F, Morrow JR Jr, Jackson AW, Sjöström M, Blair SN. Association between muscular strength and mortality in men: prospective cohort study. BMJ. 2008 Jul 1; 337:a439. PubMed PMID:18595904; PubMed Central PMCID: PMC2453303.
- Ruiz JR, Sui X, Lobelo F, Lee DC, Morrow JR Jr, Jackson AW, Hébert JR, Matthews CE, Sjöström M, Blair SN. Muscular strength and adiposity as predictors of adulthood cancer mortality in men. Cancer Epidemiol Biomarkers Prev. 2009 May; 18 (5) :1468-76. PubMed PMID:19366909.
- Rupert RL, Manello D, Sandefur R. Maintenance care: health promotion services administered to US chiropractic patients aged 65 and older, part II. J Manipulative Physiol Ther. 2000 Jan; 23 (1) :10-9. PubMed PMID:10658871.
- Ryan DH, Kushner R. The state of obesity and obesity research. JAMA. 2010 Oct 27; 304 (16) :1835-6. PubMed PMID:20935336.
- Saavedra JM, Bauman NA, Oung I, Perman JA, Yolken RH. Feeding of Bifidobacterium bifidum and Streptococcus thermophilus to infants in hospital for prevention of diarrhoea and shedding of rotavirus. Lancet. 1994 Oct 15; 344 (8929) :1046-9. PubMed PMID:7934445.
- Salli Systems Basic facts about sitting" 2004 www.salli.com

- Sampath H, Ntambi JM. Polyunsaturated fatty acid regulation of gene expression. Nutr Rev. 2004 Sep; 62 (9) :333-9. PubMed PMID:15497766.
- Samuelson RJ. Let them go bankrupt, soon Solving Social Security and Medicare. Newsweek. 2009 Jun 1; 153 (22) :23. PubMed PMID:19522176.
- Santangelo C, Varì R, Scazzocchio B, Di Benedetto R, Filesi C, Masella R. Polyphenols, intracellular signalling and inflammation. Ann Ist Super Sanita. 2007; 43 (4) :394-405. PubMed PMID:18209273.
- Sapolsky RM. Organismal stress and telomeric aging: an unexpected connection. Proc Natl Acad Sci U S A. 2004 Dec 14; 101 (50) :17323-4. PubMed PMID:15579535; PubMed Central PMCID: PMC536029.
- Sasco AJ. Epidemiology of breast cancer: an environmental disease?. APMIS. 2001 May; 109 (5) :321-32. PubMed PMID:11478680.
- Schatz IJ, Masaki K, Yano K, Chen R, Rodriguez BL, Curb JD. Cholesterol and all-cause mortality in elderly people from the Honolulu Heart Program: a cohort study. Lancet. 2001 Aug 4; 358 (9279) :351-5. PubMed PMID:11502313.
- Schlosser, E. 2002. Fast Food Nation. Houghton Miffin Company. New York, NY.
- Schmahmann JD. From movement to thought: anatomic substrates of the cerebellar contribution to cognitive processing. Hum Brain Mapp. 1996; 4 (3) :174-98. PubMed PMID:20408197.
- Schmahmann JD, Sherman JC. The cerebellar cognitive affective syndrome. Brain. 1998 Apr; 121 (Pt 4):561-79. PubMed PMID:9577385.
- Schmahmann JD, Sherman JC. Cerebellar cognitive affective syndrome. Int Rev Neurobiol. 1997; 41:433-40. PubMed PMID:9378601.
- Schmidt S. Mindfulness and healing intention: concepts, practice, and research evaluation. J Altern Complement Med. 2004; 10 Suppl 1:S7-14. PubMed PMID:15630818.
- Schulkin, J, 2004. Alostasis, Homeostasis, and the Costs of Physiological Adaptation. Cambridge University Press. New York, NY.
- Schulz LO, Bennett PH, Ravussin E, Kidd JR, Kidd KK, Esparza J, Valencia ME. Effects of traditional and western environments on prevalence of type 2 diabetes in Pima Indians in Mexico and the US.

Diabetes Care. 2006 Aug; 29 (8) :1866-71. PubMed PMID:16873794.

- Schwartzbauer et al. Athletic performance and physiological measures in baseball players following upper cervical chiropractic care: A pilot study. JVSR 1997
- Seals DR, Bell C. Chronic sympathetic activation: consequence and cause of age-associated obesity?. Diabetes. 2004 Feb; 53 (2) :276-84. PubMed PMID:14747276.
- Seaman D. Health care for our bones: a practical nutritional approach to preventing osteoporosis. J Manipulative Physiol Ther. 2004 Nov-Dec; 27 (9) :591-5. PubMed PMID:15614247.
- Seaman DR, Winterstein JF. Dysafferentation: a novel term to describe the neuropathophysiological effects of joint complex dysfunction A look at likely mechanisms of symptom generation. J Manipulative Physiol Ther. 1998 May; 21 (4) :267-80. PubMed PMID:9608382.
- Sebastian A, Frassetto LA, Sellmeyer DE, Merriam RL, Morris RC Jr. Estimation of the net acid load of the diet of ancestral preagricultural Homo sapiens and their hominid ancestors. Am J Clin Nutr. 2002 Dec; 76 (6) :1308-16. PubMed PMID:12450898.
- Seeman TE, McEwen BS, Rowe JW, Singer BH. Allostatic load as a marker of cumulative biological risk: MacArthur studies of successful aging. Proc Natl Acad Sci U S A. 2001 Apr 10; 98 (8) :4770-5. PubMed PMID:11287659; PubMed Central PMCID: PMC31909.
- Seeman TE, Singer BH, Ryff CD, Dienberg Love G, Levy-Storms L. Social relationships, gender, and allostatic load across two age cohorts. Psychosom Med. 2002 May-Jun; 64 (3) :395-406. PubMed PMID:12021414.
- Seeman TE, McEwen BS. Impact of social environment characteristics on neuroendocrine regulation. Psychosom Med. 1996 Sep-Oct; 58 (5) :459-71. PubMed PMID:8902897.
- Seitz, J.A. I move therefore I am. Psychology Today 1993; 26.
- Selye, Hans. 1984. The Stress of Life, revised edition. The McGraw-Hill Companies, Inc. New York, NY.
- Sendemir A, Sendemir E, Kosmehl H, Jirikowski GF. Expression of

sex hormone-binding globulin, oxytocin receptor, caveolin-1 and p21 in leiomyoma. Gynecol Endocrinol. 2008 Feb; 24 (2) :105-12. PubMed PMID:17952758.

- Servan-Schreiber D. 2008. Anticancer: a new way of life. Penguin Books. New York, NY.
- Shonkoff JP, Boyce WT, McEwen BS. Neuroscience, molecular biology, and the childhood roots of health disparities: building a new framework for health promotion and disease prevention. JAMA. 2009 Jun 3; 301 (21) :2252-9. PubMed PMID:19491187.
- Shortell SM. Bending the cost curve: a critical component of health care reform. JAMA. 2009 Sep 16; 302 (11) :1223-4. PubMed PMID:19755703.
- Simopoulos AP. Evolutionary aspects of diet and essential fatty acids. World Rev Nutr Diet. 2001; 88:18-27. PubMed PMID:11935953.
- Siris ES, Miller PD, Barrett-Connor E, Faulkner KG, Wehren LE, Abbott TA, Berger ML, Santora AC, Sherwood LM. Identification and fracture outcomes of undiagnosed low bone mineral density in postmenopausal women: results from the National Osteoporosis Risk Assessment. JAMA. 2001 Dec 12; 286 (22) :2815-22. PubMed PMID:11735756.
- Sloan EK, Capitanio JP, Tarara RP, Mendoza SP, Mason WA, Cole SW. Social stress enhances sympathetic innervation of primate lymph nodes: mechanisms and implications for viral pathogenesis. J Neurosci. 2007 Aug 15; 27 (33) :8857-65. PubMed PMID:17699667.
- Stewart JA. The detrimental effects of allostasis: allostatic load as a measure of cumulative stress. J Physiol Anthropol. 2006 Jan; 25 (1) :133-45. PubMed PMID:16617218.
- Stoner GD, Wang LS, Zikri N, Chen T, Hecht SS, Huang C, Sardo C, Lechner JF. Cancer prevention with freeze-dried berries and berry components. Semin Cancer Biol. 2007 Oct; 17 (5) :403-10. PubMed PMID:17574861; PubMed Central PMCID: PMC2196225.
- Strannegård O, Strannegård IL. The causes of the increasing prevalence of allergy: is atopy a microbial deprivation disorder?. Allergy. 2001 Feb; 56 (2) :91-102. PubMed PMID:11167368.
- Stumvoll M, Tataranni PA, Stefan N, Vozarova B, Bogardus C. Glucose allostasis. Diabetes. 2003 Apr; 52 (4) :903-9. PubMed PMID:12663459.

- Sturm R. Childhood obesity - what we can learn from existing data on societal trends, part 1. Prev Chronic Dis. 2005 Jan; 2 (1) :A12. PubMed PMID:15670465; PubMed Central PMCID: PMC1323315.
- Sturm R. Childhood obesity -- what we can learn from existing data on societal trends, part 2. Prev Chronic Dis. 2005 Apr; 2 (2) :A20. PubMed PMID:15888231; PubMed Central PMCID: PMC1327714.
- Sturm R, Ringel J, Andreyeva T. "Increasing Obesity Rates and Disability Trends," Health Affairs, Vol. 23, No. 2, March/April 2004, pp. 1–7.
- Suk WA, Collman GW. Genes and the environment: their impact on children's health. Environ Health Perspect. 1998 Jun; 106 Suppl 3:817-20. PubMed PMID:9646043; PubMed Central PMCID: PMC1533074.
- Swaab DF, Bao AM, Lucassen PJ. The stress system in the human brain in depression and neurodegeneration. Ageing Res Rev. 2005 May; 4 (2) :141-94. PubMed PMID:15996533.
- Sylvia LG, Ametrano RM, Nierenberg AA. Exercise treatment for bipolar disorder: potential mechanisms of action mediated through increased neurogenesis and decreased allostatic load. Psychother Psychosom. 2010; 79 (2) :87-96. PubMed PMID:20051706.
- Symons BP, Leonard T, Herzog W. Internal forces sustained by the vertebral artery during spinal manipulative therapy. J Manipulative Physiol Ther 2002;25:504-510.
- Talarovicova A, Krskova L, Kiss A. Some assessments of the amygdala role in suprahypothalamic neuroendocrine regulation: a minireview. Endocr Regul. 2007 Nov; 41 (4) :155-62. PubMed PMID:18257652.
- Tan S, Tillisch K, Mayer E. Functional Somatic Syndromes: Emerging Biomedical Models and Traditional Chinese Medicine. Evid Based Complement Alternat Med. 2004 Jun 1; 1 (1) :35-40. PubMed PMID:15257324; PubMed Central PMCID: PMC442118.
- Terrett, A.G. Cerebral dysfunction: a theory to explain some of the effects of chiropractic manipulation. Chiropractic Technique 1993; 5 (3).
- Terret et al. Manipulation and pain tolerance. American Journal of Physical Medicine 1984 63 (5).

- Thomas, JR, Nelson, JK. 1985. Introduction to Research in Health Education, Recreation and Dance. Human Kinetics Books. Champaign, IL.
- Thomas, JR, Nelson, JK. 1990. Research Methods in Physical Activity. Human Kinetics Books. Champaign, IL.
- Thürmer HL, Lund-Larsen PG, Tverdal A. Is blood pressure treatment as effective in a population setting as in controlled trials? Results from a prospective study. J Hypertens. 1994 Apr; 12 (4) :481-90. PubMed PMID:8064174.
- Torrance B, McGuire KA, Lewanczuk R, McGavock J. Overweight, physical activity and high blood pressure in children: a review of the literature. Vasc Health Risk Manag. 2007; 3 (1) :139-49. PubMed PMID:17583184; PubMed Central PMCID: PMC1994042.
- Troyanovich SJ, Harrison DE, Harrison DD. Structural rehabilitation of the spine and posture: rationale for treatment beyond the resolution of symptoms. J Manipulative Physiol Ther. 1998 Jan; 21 (1) :37-50. PubMed PMID:9467100.
- Tsigos C, Chrousos GP. Hypothalamic-pituitary-adrenal axis, neuroendocrine factors and stress. J Psychosom Res. 2002 Oct; 53 (4) :865-71. PubMed PMID:12377295.
- Tuchin PJ. The effect of chiropractic spinal manipulative therapy on salivary cortisol levels. Australas Chiropr Osteopathy. 1998 Jul;7(2):86-92. PubMed PMID: 17987159; PubMed Central PMCID: PMC2050804.
- Tunstall RJ, Mehan KA, Wadley GD, Collier GR, Bonen A, Hargreaves M, Cameron-Smith D. Exercise training increases lipid metabolism gene expression in human skeletal muscle. Am J Physiol Endocrinol Metab. 2002 Jul; 283 (1) :E66-72. PubMed PMID:12067844.
- Valentino RJ, Van Bockstaele E. Convergent regulation of locus coeruleus activity as an adaptive response to stress. Eur J Pharmacol. 2008 Apr 7; 583 (2-3) :194-203. PubMed PMID:18255055; PubMed Central PMCID: PMC2349983.
- Vastag B. Pay attention: ritalin acts much like cocaine. JAMA . 2001 Aug 22-29;286(8):905-6.
- Velicer CM, Heckbert SR, Lampe JW, Potter JD, Robertson CA, Taplin

SH. Antibiotic use in relation to the risk of breast cancer. JAMA. 2004 Feb 18; 291 (7) :827-35. PubMed PMID:14970061.

- Vieira VJ, Ronan AM, Windt MR, Tagliaferro AR. Elevated atopy in healthy obese women. Am J Clin Nutr. 2005 Sep; 82 (3) :504-9. PubMed PMID:16155260.
- Videman, T. Experimental models of osteoarthritis: the role of immobilization. Clinical Biomechanics 1987 (2)
- Villeneuve, PJ; Mao Y (November 1994). "Lifetime probability of developing lung cancer, by smoking status, Canada". Canadian Journal of Public Health 85 (6): 385–388. PMID 7895211
- Vora & Bates. The effects of spinal manipulation on the immune system (A preliminary report) The ACA Journal of Chiropractic 1980
- Wahn U. What drives the allergic march?. Allergy. 2000 Jul; 55 (7) :591-9. PubMed PMID:10921457.
- Waterland RA, Jirtle RL. Transposable elements: targets for early nutritional effects on epigenetic gene regulation. Mol Cell Biol. 2003 Aug;23(15):5293-300. PubMed PMID: 12861015; PubMed Central PMCID: PMC165709.
- Watters, Ethan. DNA is not Destiny: The New Science of Epigenetics Rewrites the Rules of Disease, Heredity, and Identity. Discover Nov 2006
- Watson DH, Trott PH. Cervical headache: an investigation of natural head posture and upper cervical flexor muscle performance. Cephalalgia. 1993 Aug; 13 (4) :272-84; discussion 232. PubMed PMID:8374943.
- Waterland RA, Jirtle RL. Early nutrition, epigenetic changes at transposons and imprinted genes, and enhanced susceptibility to adult chronic diseases. Nutrition. 2004 Jan;20(1):63-8. Review. PubMed PMID: 14698016.
- Wayne SJ, Neuhouser ML, Ulrich CM, Koprowski C, Baumgartner KB, Baumgartner RN, McTiernan A, Bernstein L, Ballard-Barbash R. Dietary fiber is associated with serum sex hormones and insulin-related peptides in postmenopausal breast cancer survivors. Breast Cancer Res Treat. 2008 Nov; 112 (1) :149-58. PubMed PMID:18058020.

- Wijndaele K, Duvigneaud N, Matton L, Duquet W, Delecluse C, Thomis M, Beunen G, Lefevre J, Philippaerts RM. Sedentary behaviour, physical activity and a continuous metabolic syndrome risk score in adults. Eur J Clin Nutr. 2009 Mar; 63 (3) :421-9. PubMed PMID:17971826.
- Wilk v. American Medical Association, (7th Cir. 1990).
- Willcox BJ, He Q, Chen R, Yano K, Masaki KH, Grove JS, Donlon TA, Willcox DC, Curb JD. Midlife risk factors and healthy survival in men. JAMA. 2006 Nov 15; 296 (19) :2343-50. PubMed PMID:17105797.
- Wilmore, JH, Costill, DL. 2004. Physiology of Sport and Ecercise, Third Edition. Human Kinetics. Champaign, IL.
- Witecki K, Czapla A, Kido⊠ Z, Pawlas K, Powazka E. The application of computer posturography in psychological diagnosis. Med Sci Monit. 2003 Dec; 9 (12) :MT133-8. PubMed PMID:14646982.
- Whittingham W, Nilsson N. Active range of motion in the cervical spine increases after spinal manipulation (toggle recoil). J Manipulative Physiol Ther. 2001 Nov-Dec;24(9):552-5. PubMed PMID: 11753327.
- Wong, William, ND, PhD. 1999. Treating Diabetes With Enzymes: What We Know Now. http://www.totalityofbeing.com/FramelessPages/Articles/TreatingDiabetes.htm
- Woolf SH. A closer look at the economic argument for disease prevention. JAMA. 2009 Feb 4; 301 (5) :536-8. PubMed PMID:19190319.
- Wright EF, Domenech MA, Fischer JR Jr. Usefulness of posture training for patients with temporomandibular disorders. J Am Dent Assoc. 2000 Feb; 131 (2) :202-10. PubMed PMID:10680388.
- Wu AH, Yu MC, Tseng CC, Stanczyk FZ, Pike MC. Diabetes and risk of breast cancer in Asian-American women. Carcinogenesis. 2007 Jul; 28 (7) :1561-6. PubMed PMID:17440036.
- Wärnberg J, Marcos A. Low-grade inflammation and the metabolic syndrome in children and adolescents. Curr Opin Lipidol. 2008 Feb; 19 (1) :11-5. PubMed PMID:18196981.
- Yates LB, Djoussé L, Kurth T, Buring JE, Gaziano JM. Exceptional longevity in men: modifiable factors associated with survival and function to age 90 years. Arch Intern Med. 2008 Feb 11; 168 (3) :284-90.

PubMed PMID:18268169.

- Yates RG, Lamping DL, Abram NL, Wright C. Effects of chiropractic treatment on blood pressure and anxiety: a randomized, controlled trial. J Manipulative Physiol Ther. 1988 Dec; 11 (6) :484-8. PubMed PMID:3075649.
- Young, Robert PhD & Young, Shelley The pH Miracle. Warner Books, New York 2002
- Zhang, J. The effects of chiropractic care on short-term power spectrum analysis of heart rate variability. JVSR 1998
- Zeginiadou T, Kortsaris AH, Koliais S, Antonoglou O. Sex hormone binding globulin inhibits strongly the uptake of estradiol by human breast carcinoma cells via a deprivative mechanism. Cancer Biochem Biophys. 1998 Oct; 16 (3) :253-63. PubMed PMID:10072209.

Index

A

B

C

D

E

F

G

H

I

L

N

O

O

P

R

S

T

V

W

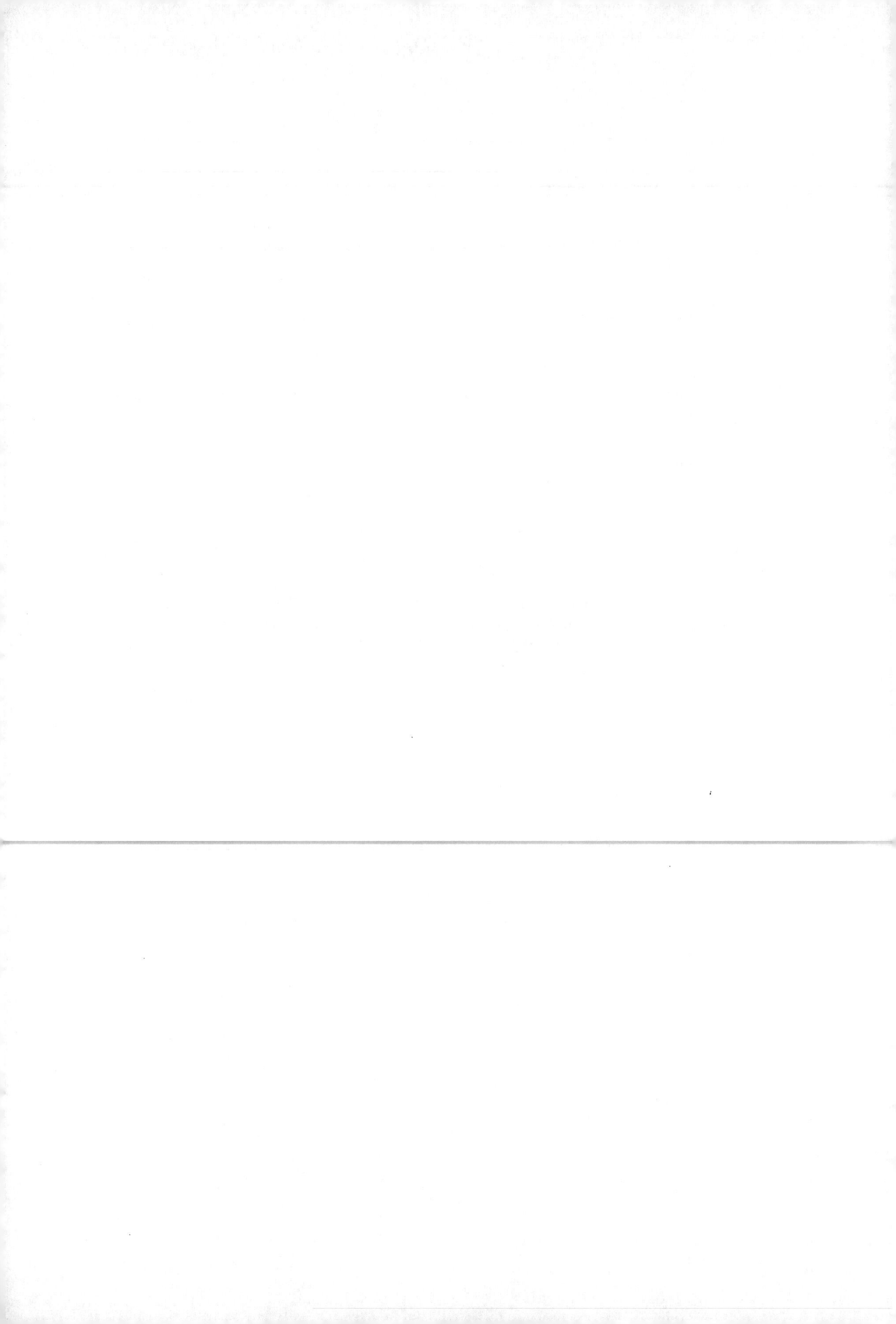